The Creative Dukan Diet

A Convenient Way to Start and Manage Your Diet

BY: Ivy Hope

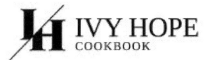

Copyright/License Page

Table of Contents

Introduction

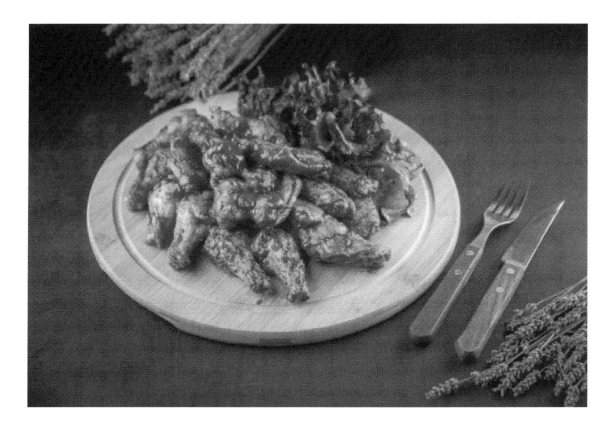

The Dukan Diet is a strict low-carbohydrate diet which is ideally suited for both the average person, as well those suffering from a variety of health conditions.

Now coming to specific benefits associated with the Dukan Diet, there is no doubt that it works very well as far as targeting overweight and obesity are concerned. The first phase itself works very well and many people who diet say that they have lost quite a few pounds (provided they have followed the program correctly).

There is another important point to be kept in mind while following this diet. You are not supposed to count your calorie intake during the first few phases because mentally, it might start boring you, and your commitment levels might start fading in this phase. It is always advisable to simply go by what the diet program says rather than trying to measure the calories which you are eating.

It is extremely important that you drink at least the recommended 1.5 to 3 quarts of water each day to keep your kidneys flushed out, as the high amounts of protein you are going to be eating might cause the build-up of uric acid. This could be a problem for those people with a family history of gout.

The water will also help you avoid another common problem that occurs on the Dukan Diet when people neglect to consume the required amount of oat bran, namely, constipation.

You may go through some withdrawal symptoms as you go "cold-turkey" and stop eating carbohydrates. These might include flu-like symptoms of headache, fever, chills, dizziness, weakness, fatigue and nausea. These symptoms usually pass in 3-5 days.

The Dukan diet protocol has a specific list of allowed foods thereby eliminating carbs completely. Moreover, it is the only diet protocol that is based on a four-phase program, wherein progress is accelerated and losses are maximized.

The Dukan Diet Phases

Here, each of the phases of the Dukan diet will be extensively discussed for better execution of the diet after gaining a thorough understanding.

Attack Phase

The attack phase aims to jumpstart the body into losing weight fast. It usually lasts for 1-5 days, depending on your current weight. It may also vary since everybody is different and may take longer or shorter depending on the person's metabolism. A calculator online is readily available in order for you to calculate your true weight and gauge the exact time to stop the attack phase. To illustrate if your excess body weight is:

10 pounds or less = 1 to 2 days

15-30 pounds = 3 to 5 days

40 pounds and above = 7 days (please consult your physician before proceeding)

This phase may be the hardest to accomplish since its goal is to establish eating habits that do not include starchy and unhealthy foods. This is also that part of the Dukan Diet wherein you would lose the greatest amount of weight. The greatest enemies in this phase are the hunger cravings from a carbohydrate-rich diet and also the old eating habits that you had for years.

What is crucial in a protein diet is water intake. Every day, you must drink at least 1.5 liters of water in order to avoid dehydration and overworking of the kidneys. At the start of the Dukan Diet, you will learn to incorporate 1.5 tablespoons of oat bran in your food. You may mix it in your food and prepare it in any way you want. The oat bran will provide the fiber that you will need in this phase. You can eat any amount of food as long as it is allowed in the food list and prepared in an acceptable manner. Only 68 of the various protein sources are allowed in this phase.

Heavy exercise is a no-no in this phase. This is a time when your body is still adjusting to the new eating habits that you are forming. Rigorous and long periods of exercise are not advised, but a 20-minute light to moderate amount of exercise would be recommended.

Do not be discouraged if you lose less than what you expect; each of us has a different body, and results will differ. Just be diligent in following the regime, and you may achieve the excellent results that you deserve.

Cruise Phase

This is the part when you slowly reintroduce other forms of food such as vegetables and fruits. In this phase, you will have more choices in food. The goal of this phase is to continue with a steady amount of weight loss until you reach your desired weight. You will lose only about 1 -2 pounds every 3 days, comparatively lower than in the first phase.

The weight loss in this phase is slow and gradual. The aim here is to lose the stubborn fats left behind while maintaining your lean body mass. In the attack phase, you are allowed to eat 68 different protein sources; in this case, 32 vegetables are added. The meals in this phase are protein and non-starchy vegetables. You can also increase your oat bran intake to 2 tablespoons daily. Similar to the attack phase, you should consume 1.5 liters of water every day or more to keep you hydrated.

The level of activity is also the same, but you can increase the duration to 30 minutes. Since your body is getting used to the new eating habits, you can endure a longer work-out routine.

Consolidation Phase

Congratulations! You have truly succeeded in achieving your desired weight. Though you have succeeded, there is also an emerging problem once you reach this phase. How can you prevent gaining back the weight that you lost? This is the phase that will help you prevent the pounds from creeping back. An excellent diet should provide the ways to ensure the healthy and sexy new you is here to stay.

Several foods that were forbidden in the previous 2 phases are now being brought back on the menu. You will have more variety in preparing your food. You will be allowed to eat cheese, bread, and starchy foods such as potatoes. You will be allowed to have celebration meals in this phase by having wine and cakes. The first half of the consolidation phase will be more restricted and is only allowed a single celebration meal a week. More foods that are restricted in the first half of the third phase will be added in proportions.

But you have to keep in mind to eat the foods that are healthy and natural. It is best to consume foods that are not processed since processed foods contain sugar and preservatives that are bad for your health. You can eat ice cream and pizza but not on a regular basis. Always remember that eating well is a lifelong commitment. In every week in the consolidation phase, you will have a day of eating only pure protein or preferably called PP Thursday by Dukan dieters.

The rule in this phase is that for every pound that you lost since the beginning, you need to be in the consolidation phase for five days. If you lose 10 pounds, you will be in the consolidation phase for 50 days. This rule is easy to understand and remember.

Maintaining physical activity is crucial to keeping the weight off. Similar to the cruise phase, you are allowed to engage in physical exercises for around 30 minutes. Always listen to your body; if you think you can't do it, don't force yourself.

Stabilization Phase

The final phase of the Dukan diet is the stabilization phase in which the dieter has gained liberty in choosing her/his own food. The common problem with general dieters is that when they reach their goal weight, they get back to their old eating habits. This is also a problem with several other diets as those diets only cater to losing weight and not keeping them off for a lifetime.

This phase is a permanent and life-long process to prevent you from gaining the pounds again. There are only three simple rules to follow:

1. Increase your oat bran consumption to 3 tablespoons per day.

2. Take a day with only pure protein. You may still follow the consolidation phase's PP Thursday or Pure Protein Thursday.

3. Exercise according to what your body can. You may have a rigorous exercise as long as you do not overexert yourself.

You will only need to remember these things to keep your weight and stay slim and healthy and enjoy your life ahead.

Pros and Cons of the Dukan Diet

Pros of the diet

Weight loss

Weight loss is one of the biggest advantages of the Dukan diet. The diet is designed to help obese people lose weight and also focuses on not allowing that weight to be regained. The diet thereby helps you cut down on the risk of developing obesity related diseases such as heart diseases, hypertension, high blood pressure, diabetes type II, etc.

No muscle loss

Since the main nutrient in focus during the diet is "protein", muscle loss will not be a problem. Protein is the main element responsible for developing and maintaining healthy muscles.

No calorie counting

Unlike other diets, the Dukan diet does not stress calorie counting. Several diets require the dieter to completely measure out everything that they eat like in the zone diet. That becomes extremely tedious and might force a person to give up midway. That danger is avoided in the Dukan diet.

No portion control

The diet does not restrict the amount of food that can be consumed. It is important to eat foods that are only mentioned in the phase wise food list, but there is no restriction on how much of those foods can be consumed, which makes it ideal for people who are used to consuming large portions.

Easy to follow

The diet is not rocket science. It is quite easy to understand and follow. It clearly specifies the four different phases and their rules and also gives you an exhaustive food-list to choose from. It does not get any easier than that folks!

Result oriented

The diet is extremely result oriented and within one or two weeks, you start to notice a loss in your weight. The weight loss is progressive, and month after month, you will feel lighter and lighter until you reach your ideal weight.

Meats encouraged

The diet mainly focuses on the consumption of lean meats which is great news for meat lovers. As we all know, meat is extremely rich in proteins, and since that is the main nutrient in focus in the diet, it works out to be the most efficient and feasible form of ingredient for the diet.

Celebratory meals

The 2 celebratory meals that are allowed from the consolidation phase onwards are the highlight of the diet. The two meals serve as great relief especially for people who are accustomed to a diet rich in junk food. The meals are rightfully named as "celebration meals."

Sweeteners

The diet does not restrict the consumption of artificial sweeteners and diet sodas. Dukan dieters can consume sweetener based dishes and also drink diet soda to their liking. The sweeteners can be used for desserts.

Vegetarian-friendly

The diet also encourages the consumption of vegetarian food substances with a substantial amount of choice for vegetarians. Although not as much variety as is available for non-vegetarians, there is enough choice of vegetables and meat substitutes like tofu for the vegetarians.

Cons of the diet

<u>Deficiencies</u>

The diet causes several nutrient deficiencies especially during the attack phase. Since the main focus is proteins, vitamins such as A, D, C and E are not incorporated, which can cause bone loss. There is also the lack of iron which can cause temporary loss of hair and brittle nails etc. Doctor Dukan recommends the consumption of nutritional supplements to combat this very problem.

<u>Not for vegans</u>

The diet is not ideal for vegans since there is a lot of consumption of meat and the food-lists do not contain any vegan friendly foods. But in the argument of the diet, vegans do not necessarily require weight loss regimes, and it is safe to say that vegans are therefore not included in the diet.

<u>Fatigue</u>

Fatigue is tiredness that can arise out of the nutrient restrictions in the diet. Carbohydrates are important for energy upkeep, and the lack of the nutrient can cause a dieter to face mood swings and pangs of fatigue.

<u>Sweeteners and sodas</u>

The diet does allow for artificial sweeteners and soda to be consumed and can be counted as a plus, but on the flip side, these are not necessarily healthy choices and can, in fact, counteract the goodness that the diet provides.

Bad breath

Bad breath is a major cause of concern for the diet. The high protein intake can also cause flatulence and leave behind a metallic taste in the mouth. The problem of bad breath is strongest during the attack phase.

Kidney damage

The consistent burning of body fat as opposed to calories causes the kidneys and liver to take on an additional burden, which can result in severe damage in due course. The excess load can cause the urine to darken and emit an acrid odor.

Withdrawal symptoms

Once the diet is completed, withdrawal symptoms can set in. These symptoms can be the likes of fatigue, nausea and headaches as the body goes through a lot of change and will find it difficult to go back to the previous type of diet.

Expensive

The diet can turn out to be an expensive affair; lean meats can be quite costly. The diet also requires you to consume nutritional supplements which add to the costs. The diet will easily make you shell out a few hundred dollars more every month.

High cholesterol

The excessive consumption of meat can cause a surge in your level of cholesterol. Despite being lean, all meats contain some amount of fat, and that fat can build up over time to block the arteries. The diet is, therefore, also not suitable for people with high levels of cholesterol.

Exercise

The diet inter-depends on exercise to a large extent. Exercising is not a convenient option for many people, and the interdependency makes it difficult for these people to see a substantial result. Right from the attack phase to the last phase, dieters are required to exercise on a daily basis.

Gout and constipation

People on high protein diets are extremely likely to develop gout. Gout is a condition wherein inflammatory arthritis can attack the limbs. The lack of fiber in the diet can cause extreme constipation owing to which a person has to compulsorily drink at least 9-10 glasses of water a day especially during the attack phase.

Food to Avoid

Because the Dukan Diet excludes calorie-rich fats, weight loss is maximized. The flavor that is lost by eating lean meat can be made up for by experimenting with spices, lemon juice, soy sauce, and other marinades to make your meals healthy and delicious.

Dukan Diet excludes processed foods and drinks, which eliminates unhealthy preservatives from the diet. Pre-made or frozen meals often contain added sugar or salt for flavor, so eliminating them from the diet is beneficial for the heart and will result in weight loss. Even processed foods that seem healthy, like juice, are filled with extra sugar and contain none of the filling fiber of whole, raw fruit. There is just no way to know what has been added into frozen TV dinners. When you are on the Dukan Diet, you will eat only whole, natural foods that you can list all the ingredients to.

The most obvious and drastic element of the Dukan Diet is the lack of carbohydrates. Grains and starches are calorie-dense, easy to digest, and lack vitamins. Because they are so easy to digest, our body does so quickly, causing our blood sugar to rise sharply. This is why carbs are a source of quick energy, but what happens next will often result in an unhealthy energy crash. After the blood sugar spikes, our bodies will then respond by quickly producing the hormone insulin to help digest the carbs. This results in a low feeling, mental fogginess, and lack of fullness, causing us to eat more to feel full again. On the Dukan Diet, the protein and fiber-dense foods will keep you fuller longer, meaning you will have no need to count calories to make sure you don't overeat. Fortunately, the Dukan Diet offers an alternative to carbs with Shirataki noodles that have barely any calories at all.

Many people don't realize it, but dairy is packed with fat and sugars. Dairy can often cause breakouts or digestive problems in adults, so reducing or eliminating it from the diet can result in healthier skin and more regular digestion. With the Dukan Diet, low or no fat dairy that is low in sugar is okay in moderation.

The Dukan Diet also excludes fruit in the first two phases. While it is true that fruit contains fiber and vitamins, they don't have anything that can't be found in the vegetables and goji berries on the allowed foods list. Goji berries are rich in 11 different kinds of vitamins, and many of the vegetables on the list such as kale, spinach, and celery are packed with fiber. Like protein, fiber is a dense food that will keep you full longer and reduce cravings.

Of course, the Dukan Diet eliminates sweets like cookies and chocolate in the first two phases as these items are calorie dense, fatty, and have no nutritional value. Don't worry; you'll will be able to eat them again in the final two phases, but in limited portions.

The Dukan diet helps you lose weight in several ways. You eat less because:

- You are not as hungry due to the appetite suppressant effect that protein has.

- You can resist unhealthy foods because you are satiated.

- Your body is forced to burn calories on a high protein diet differently because your diet only contains 1 of the 3 nutrient categories.

- Excess water is flushed out of your body instead of being retained and accumulating.

- Your body burns more calories because it must work harder just to digest and extract calories from the proteins that you consume.

- You are eating natural foods instead of processed foods high in additives and other unwanted compounds.

Frequently Asked Questions

1) Am I allowed to consume any quantity of food?

Yes, you are allowed to consume any quantity of protein-rich food. However, there is a restriction on the number of eggs you can consume. You are only allowed to consume two eggs with yolk during the week and unlimited egg whites.

2) Can I consume lentils and split peas on protein days?

Split peas aren't allowed until the third phase (consolidation phase). Two tablespoons of lentils per day are allowed on pure protein days (only if you are a vegan or vegetarian).

3) Can I consume alcohol when on the diet?

No alcohol until the third phase (consolidation phase).

4) What are the beverages I am allowed?

You can drink both iced and hot coffee and tea without sugar. You can drink milk and other dairy beverages as long as they are fat-free, low-carb and have low sugar. Calorie-free and sugar-free diet sodas and beverages are allowed. Club soda, sparkling water or seltzer can also be consumed.

5) Can I snack between my meals?

You are allowed to eat an unlimited number of snacks as long as the ingredients are within the approved 100-food list.

6) Are carrots and beets allowed in this diet?

Though both these root vegetables are well known for their sugar content, in reality, they don't contain a high amount of sugar. However, the sugar in the vegetables can be absorbed by your body and transferred to the bloodstream especially when they are cooked. You can eat these vegetables as long as you don't cook with added fat, dressing or sauce.

7) I seem to have trouble sleeping since the time I started with the diet. Is there a reason why?

Though there is no direct connection between insomnia and Dukan Diet, we have heard this complaint from most of the dieters. Consuming a lot of coffee, tea and other caffeine-rich beverages can be the reason. Your body is more sensitive to caffeine since you are consuming fewer carbs. It is therefore advised to go for decaffeinated versions of beverages. If you are really addicted to coffee and tea, try reducing the amount to take in daily.

Breakfast Recipes

Sticking to a given diet can be quite a huge task to perform especially when you encounter meals that are not properly chosen for you. However, in this section, we will highlight the best breakfast meals that are easy to prepare. Most of them have easily accessible essential ingredients just to ensure that you don't go through a hard time preparing the delicacies. Furthermore, the recipes are specially chosen to fit the needs of anyone keen on observing the Dukan diet.

Chicken Meatballs

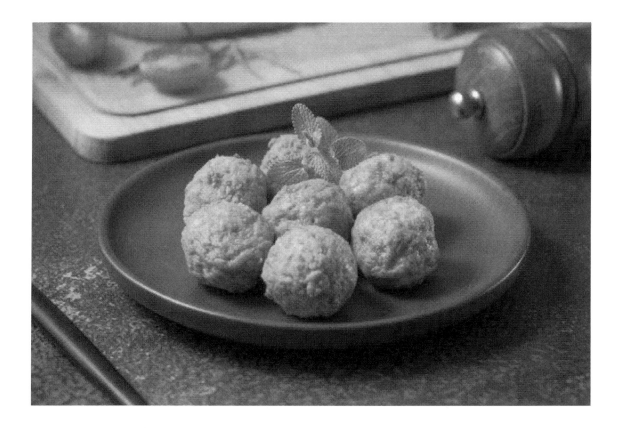

Setting a bowl of these meatballs before your dining table simply means that your family members and friends are expecting the best starter for the day. The taste of them will keep them yearning for more. The meatballs are lighter with a mouth-watering taste.

Servings: 2

Cook time: 20 minutes

Ingredients:

- 3 tbsp. chopped dill or parsley
- **Spices:** kosher salt, ground pepper and garlic powder
- 1 chopped onion, small
- 1 minced garlic clove, small
- 1 lb. chicken, ground
- 1 egg, large
- 2 tbsp. bran, oat

Directions:

1) Preheat oven to 350F.

2) Mince garlic and onion.

3) Add all ingredients to large bowl. Mix them together well.

4) Form the mixture into 15 to 20 balls and place on a pan.

5) Bake in the middle rack of 350F oven for 18-20 minutes, till juices are running clear.

6) Remove from oven and serve.

Zucchini Lasagna

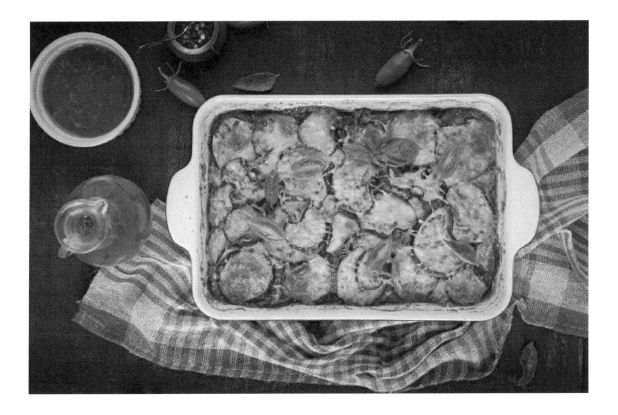

Preparing lasagna with the incorporation of at least some zucchini can be quite fun. The outcome is a low carb meal that is so delicious. The zucchini lasagna entails the incorporation of a range of veggies just to add some minerals to the taste.

Servings: 4

Cook time: 55 minutes

Ingredients:

- 1 garlic clove
- Oregano, chives, parsley, kosher salt and
- 2 lengthwise-sliced zucchinis, medium
- 2 peeled, de-seeded tomatoes, ripe, large
- 7 oz. ground beef, lean
- 3 ½ oz. mozzarella cheese, light
- 1 tbsp. tomato extract, pure
- ½ onion, medium
- 3 ½ oz. turkey breast, smoked
- Ground pepper

Directions:

1) Grill each side of sliced zucchinis in non-stick pan. Set aside.

2) Sauté onion and garlic in pan on low heat. Add kosher salt, ground pepper and beef. Cook on low.

3) Pour 1 ¾ oz. of filtered water in food processor. Add chives, parsley and tomatoes (diced). Combine till smooth.

4) Add sauce to beef. Add tomato extract. Boil mixture for 12-15 minutes.

5) Add some sauce to baking dish/pizza form for oven cooking. Form layers using zucchini, then turkey breast, then cheese and sauce. Repeat layers two times. Top with cheese and oregano.

6) Place in oven for 20-25 minutes. Then turn oven to off. Allow lasagna to sit for 12-15 minutes. Serve.

Scallops in Ham Wrap

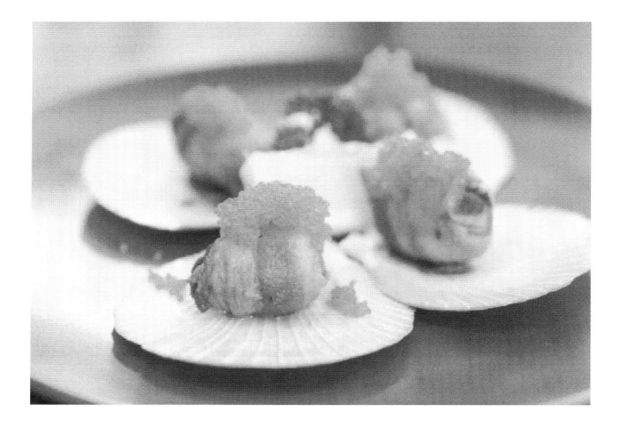

Preparing wraps of scallions in bacon can serve as a perfect way of starting your day. However, it demands a special set of ingredients such as prosciutto to make everything fine. The outcome is a meal loaded with notable meat flavors as well as the sweetness of the scallops.

Servings: 8

Cook time: 10 minutes

Ingredients:

- 4 oz. prosciutto, sliced thinly
- 2 tbsp. oil, olive
- 3 tbsp. wine, white
- ¼ tsp. pepper, black, ground
- 1 lb. scallops, large

Directions:

1) Wrap the scallops in thin prosciutto slices. Secure them with toothpicks.

2) Heat oil in large sized skillet on med-high. Place scallops in pan. Then, cook for two or three minutes per side. Season both sides with the pepper while they cook.

3) Once both sides are fried, sprinkle wine over them. Cook for one or two additional minutes.

4) Remove scallops from pan. Then, allow to drain on plate lined with paper towels. When cooled a bit, transfer them to tray. Remove toothpicks and serve.

General Tso's Chicken

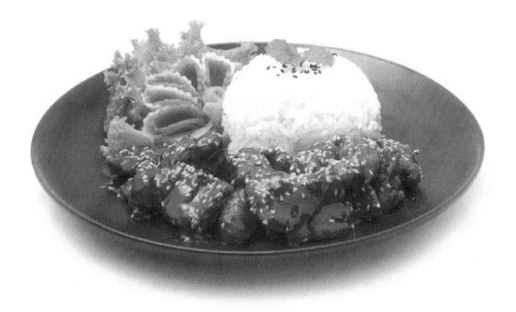

If you have never had a trial of this meal, be the first one in your home. There is no need to overburden yourself or spend much on the takeout chicken while you can make General Tso's chicken at home. Prepare it for yourself and carry it to your work area. Ensure friends enjoy the delicious taste too.

Servings: 2

Cook time: 15 minutes

Ingredients:

- Non-stick spray
- 10 oz. bite-size cut chicken breast, skinless, boneless
- 5 de-seeded, rinsed, dried chilies, red
- 1 minced garlic clove
- 2 stalks green onion, only the white part, cut small
- ½ tbsp. wine, Shaoxing
- 1 pinch salt, kosher
- 1/3 c. corn starch
- Tso sauce, bottled
- 3 minced slices ginger, peeled

Directions:

1) Marinate chicken meat in kosher salt and Shaoxing wine for 12 to 15 minutes.

2) Generously coat chicken with corn starch. Heat non-stick pan. Fry chicken till it turns lighter brown. Remove chicken using strainer. Drain off excess fat onto paper towels.

3) Heat up skillet with 1 1/2 tbsp. of non-stick spray. Add chilies, ginger and garlic into skillet. Stir fry till you can easily smell the chilies' aroma.

4) Pour tso sauce into skillet. When it thickens and boils, add chicken. Combine by stirring with sauce. Add green onions. Stir several times. Serve hot in individual dishes.

Dukan Chili

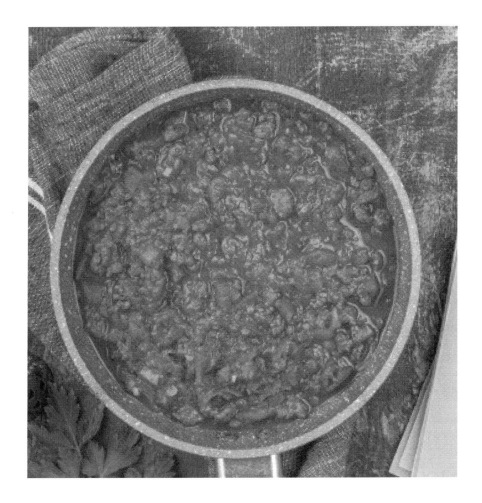

If you have been trying out the best breakfast recipes, then the Dukan Chili shouldn't miss in your list of starter meals. Each bite is tasty with the feel of cumin, chili and some little beef. You can enjoy it along with friends and family members.

Servings: 6

Cook time: 55 minutes

Ingredients:

- 1 c. cheddar cheese shreds
- 1 can undrained pinto beans
- 1 c. chopped bell pepper, green
- 7 oz. broth, beef
- 1 chopped and de-seeded jalapeno
- 1 tbsp. garlic, chopped
- 2 tbsp. chili powder
- 2 tbsp. Worcestershire sauce
- 1 ½ tsp. cumin, ground
- 1 can undrained tomatoes, diced
- 1 tsp. paprika, smoked
- 1 ½ lb. chuck, ground
- 1 can undrained kidney beans
- 1 tsp. salt, kosher
- ½ tsp. pepper, ground
- 6 oz. tomato paste
- 1 ½ lb. onions, chopped

Directions:

1) Cook the ground chuck, onions, bell peppers, garlic and jalapeno in large sized pan on med-high heat for 8-10 minutes. Crumble beef as you cook. It should not be pink at all when you're done. Stir the mixture occasionally and drain.

2) Add tomato paste, kosher salt, ground pepper, paprika, cumin and chili powder. Cook for a couple minutes until they are fragrant.

3) Add in and stir the Worcestershire sauce, undrained tomatoes and beans. Bring to boil and reduce heat. Cover and simmer for 40-45 minutes, while you occasionally stir the mixture. Serve with the cheese.

Cheese and Garlic Chicken Pocket

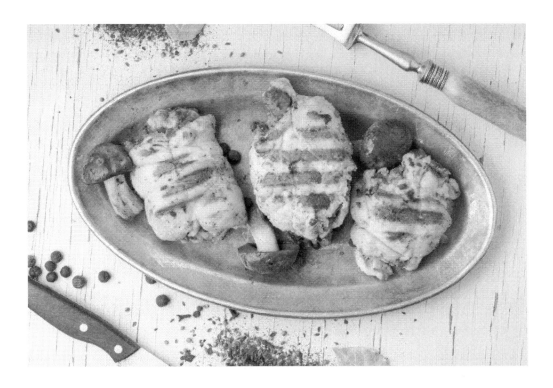

This is such a yummy recipe, and it's fairly easy to make, too. My whole family loves it, even the younger children. It's more enjoyable to make recipes that you know everyone will love.

Servings: 2

Cook time: 45 minutes

Ingredients:

- Garlic powder
- 2 chicken breasts
- Salt, kosher
- 4 tbsp. fat-free cream cheese

Directions:

1) Preheat oven to 350F.

2) Slice chicken breasts in middle area. Create pockets. Don't slice completely through.

3) Sprinkle garlic powder and kosher salt as desired inside pockets created in step 2.

4) Spread aluminum foil in roasting tray. It should be of sufficient size to put chicken breasts inside and wrap meat.

5) Place 1 to 2 tbsp. of cream cheese in pockets. Add additional garlic powder, if desired. Seal meat up using your fingers. Sprinkle parsley over the top.

6) Cover all with foil and close it up. Cook in 350F oven for 1/2 hour.

7) Open foil. Set oven to grill. Cook for 10 to 15 more minutes and serve.

Cheesy Broccoli Casserole

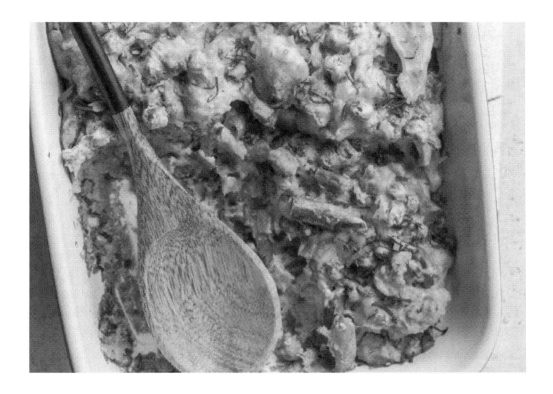

This mouth-watering delicacy would be fine if served along with a meal of your choice. If you are a lover of the green bean casserole, it is definite that you will love the Cheesy Broccoli casserole. Only a slight change is evident, a swap between green beans and broccoli. It is done to make it tastier. Don't forget the cheesy feel too.

Servings: 15

Cook time: 42 minutes

Ingredients:

- 6 oz. crispy fried onions
- 2 c. cheddar cheese shreds
- 1 c. milk
- ½ tsp. pepper, black, ground
- 10 oz. cream of mushroom soup, condensed
- 2 lb. cooked to tender-crisp, well-drained broccoli florets

Directions:

1) Preheat the oven to 350F. Mix the milk, pepper and soup in a large sized bowl.

2) Add 1 cup fried onions, 1 cup of cheese and the broccoli. Toss and coat gently.

3) Spoon the mixture in 9x13" greased baking dish. Cover dish with aluminum foil.

4) Bake for ½ hour. Remove the foil and stir fully. Sprinkle on the rest of the fried onions and cheese.

5) Leave uncovered and bake for 5-12 minutes, till onions become a golden brown and the cheese gets bubbly. Serve.

Super Breakfast Smoothie

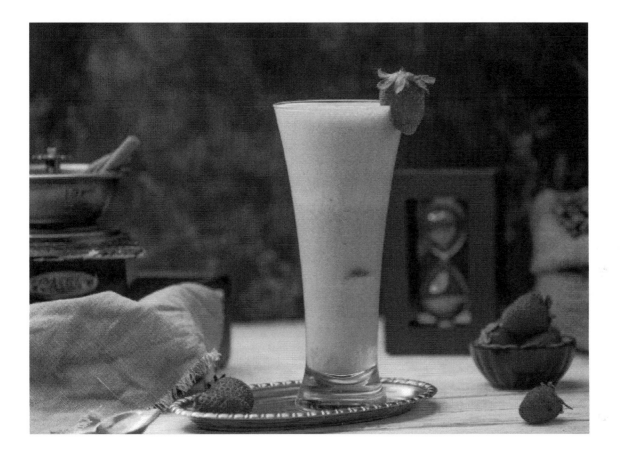

Starting your day in style requires a perfect choice of a breakfast smoothie. The super breakfast smoothie will energize you and get you ready for the day's tasks. It is loaded with lots of essential mineral components including minerals and vitamins.

Servings: 2

Cook time: 5 minutes

Ingredients:

- ½ c. strawberries, frozen and whole
- 1 c. milk, fat-free
- 1 packet milk chocolate instant breakfast mix
- 6 oz. yogurt, strawberry

Directions:

1) Place all the ingredients in food processor. Blend for a minute till smooth.

2) Serve.

Dukan Lime-Kissed Shrimp

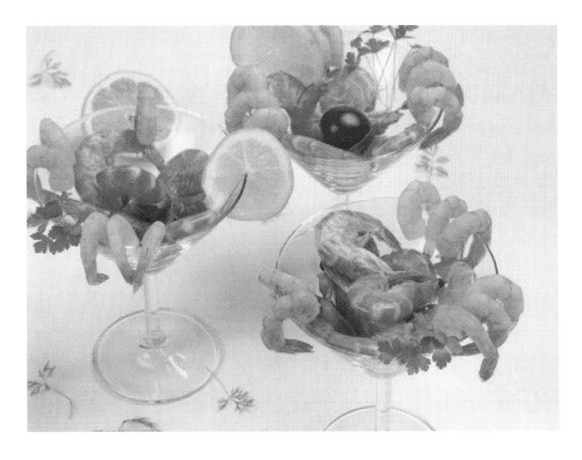

A range of flavors incorporated in a single breakfast meal can be quite good. The shrimp and lime flavors work perfectly well together and will leave tongues wagging and needing more. It requires a period of one hour to get everything done.

Servings: 2

Cook time: 25 minutes

Ingredients:

- ¾ tsp. pepper, black, ground
- 28 ready-to-cook shrimp, large
- 2 dashes salt, kosher
- Non-stick spray
- 2 tbsp. chopped onion
- ½ juiced lime

Directions:

1) Spray a skillet with non-stick spray. Heat it over med. heat.

2) Add the ingredients. Cook till onions and shrimp are done. Serve.

Chicken Marsala

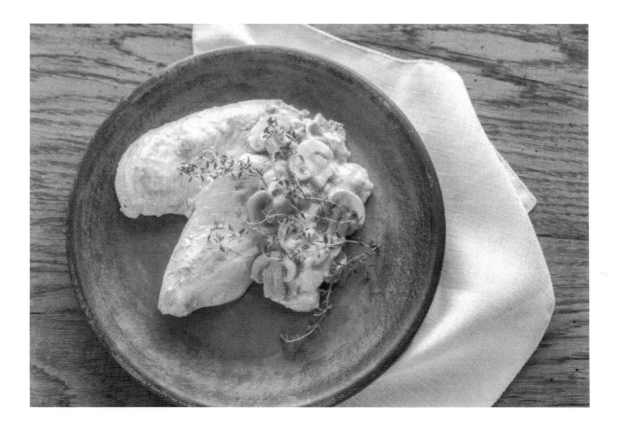

Among the quickest breakfast meals you can ever think of preparing is the Chicken Marsala. Its preparation is as simple as any other. Some of the key ingredients are boneless chicken breasts. You can try it out as it serves pretty well for family gatherings and other special occasions.

Servings: 1

Cook time: 10 minutes

Ingredients:

- 1 handful mushrooms
- 1 tbsp. garlic powder
- 1 chicken breast
- 1/3 of 1 small onion, red
- 2 tbsp. milk, skim
- 1 tbsp. curry powder
- 3 tbsp. garam masala (Middle Eastern spice mix)

Directions:

1) Butterfly-cut chicken thinly, so it cooks quicker. Add curry powder and garlic salt on each side of chicken.

2) Use oven or grill to cook chicken till both sides are brown.

3) As chicken cooks, slice mushrooms and onions into pieces of 1/2-inch or so. Add to sauté pan.

4) As the mushrooms start shrinking, add milk. Turn heat down. Allow to simmer for about five more minutes.

5) Place chicken on plates and spread the onion and mushroom mixture over the top. Serve.

Spinach Pie

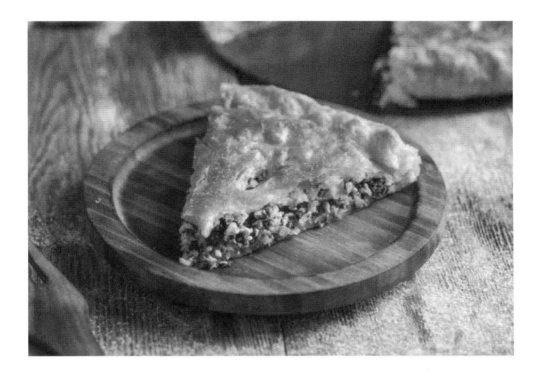

To get your breakfast within a period of 20 minutes is just amazing. Furthermore, the Spinach Pie comes with a range of flavors and tastes to enjoy. With frozen spinach, you can prepare the meal easily and enjoy it along with fellows.

Servings: 2

Cook time: 45 minutes

Ingredients:

- 1 handful basil leaves, chopped
- Black pepper, ground
- 1 handful tomatoes, cherry
- 2 beaten eggs, large
- Salt, kosher
- 8 ¾ oz. ricotta cheese, fat-free
- 2 ½ oz. fat-free cheese, feta
- 8 ¾ oz. chopped spinach, frozen
- ½ tsp. nutmeg, ground

Directions:

1) Preheat oven to 325F.

2) Thaw the spinach in your microwave oven. Squeeze it and drain water.

3) Mix ricotta cheese with kosher salt, ground pepper, basil, nutmeg, spinach and eggs in large sized bowl. Combine well.

4) Spray baking dish with oil. Pour in spinach mixture. Spread till even.

5) Garnish with halved cherry tomatoes. Sprinkle with cheese around tomatoes.

6) Place dish in oven. Cook for 35 to 40 minutes, until mixture has set well.

7) During last 5 cooking minutes, place dish under grill to brown tomatoes and cheese. Serve warm. It can also be served cold if you prefer.

Basil Thai Chicken

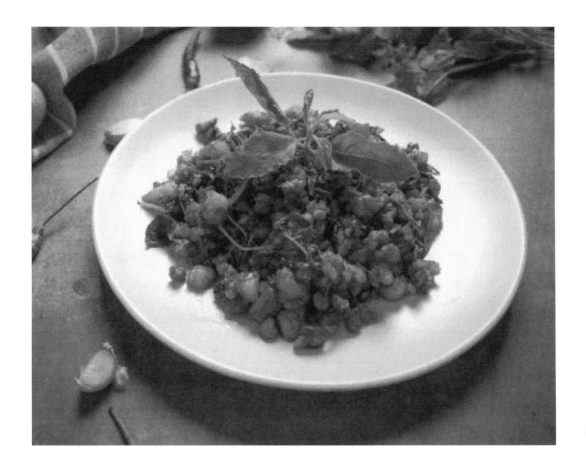

Thai dishes can be prepared in various versions. But the Basil Thai Chicken is the Dukan version of the meal, and you can be sure of enjoying it. With the use of basil alongside other better ingredients, you can be sure that your children will keep yearning for more.

Servings: 2

Cook time: 20 minutes

Ingredients:

- 4 minced garlic cloves
- 1 pinch pepper, white
- Large bunch stem-removed Thai basil, sweet
- 2 slivered lime leaves, kaffir
- 3 tsp. soy sauce, sweet, black
- 6 chopped, pounded bird (Thai) chilies
- 2 eggs, large
- ½ lb. cubed chicken, boneless
- 2 diced shallots
- 1 tbsp. fish sauce, Thai
- Non-stick spray
- 2 tsp. Splenda

Directions:

1) Spray heated skillet, then add shallots and garlic. Stir fry them till they are aromatic.

2) Add chicken meat. Stir fry quickly. Break chicken meat into small sized lumps.

3) When chicken has changed color, add chilies and seasonings. Continue stir-frying.

4) Add basil leaves. Stir a few times till basil leaves wilt and you smell their exotic fragrance.

5) Sprinkle 2 dashes of white pepper powder in mixture. Stir one last time. Transfer to dishes. Serve promptly.

Roasted Brussels Sprouts

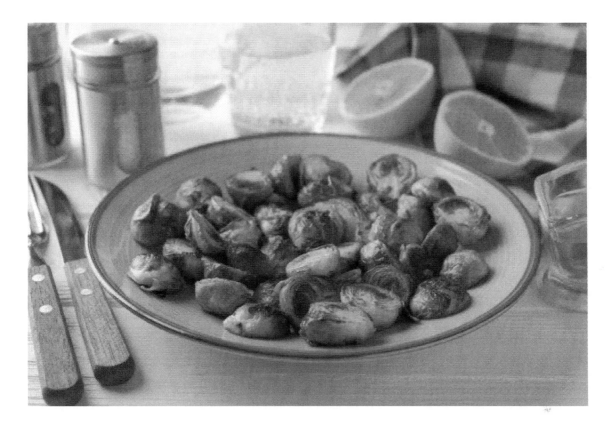

A few minutes are enough to get the best roasted Brussels sprouts. When roasted in a combination of proper and essential ingredients like honey and balsamic, you can be sure of this tasty and delicious meal. Both frozen and fresh Brussels Sprouts are better substitutes for each other.

Servings: 4

Cook time: 20 minutes

Ingredients:

- ¼ tsp. pepper, black
- 2 tbsp. vinegar, balsamic
- 2 tsp. honey, organic
- 3 tbsp. oil, olive
- 1 ½ lb. Brussels sprouts, frozen
- ½ tsp. salt, kosher

Directions:

1) Preheat the oven to 425F. Line a large sized cookie sheet with baking paper.

2) Trim ends from Brussels sprouts. Peel off any wilted leaves and toss them.

3) Arrange the Brussels sprouts on a cookie sheet. Use oil to drizzle. Season using kosher salt and ground pepper. Toss and coat the sprouts evenly. Spread them out into one layer with no pieces overlapping.

4) Roast the Brussels sprouts for 15-20 minutes, till the edges are caramelized. Remove them from the oven.

5) Whisk vinegar and honey together in a small sized bowl. Pour this mixture over the roasted Brussels sprouts. Evenly coat by tossing and serve promptly.

Dukan Moussaka

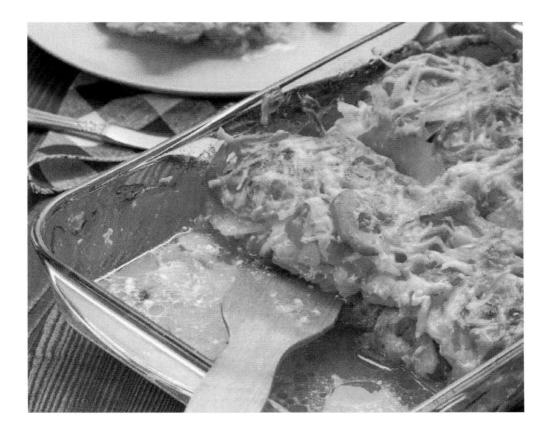

Your kids also need to enjoy and be part of active breakfast meals. With the inclusion of various essential ingredients, Dukan Moussaka is just the best for the health needs of your child and yourself.

Servings: 5

Cook time: 1 hour 30 minutes

Ingredients:

- ½ c. bran, oat
- 1 can tomatoes, diced
- 3 tbsp. grated Parmesan cheese
- 1 dash nutmeg, ground
- 2 lb. beef, ground
- 1 onion, chopped
- 2 tbsp. oregano, dried
- 2 sliced eggplants, large
- Chopped parsley, fresh
- 1 c. wine, red
- 1 tsp. cinnamon, ground
- 2 eggs, large

For the sauce

- 1 dash nutmeg and cinnamon
- 2 tbsp. Milk
- 3 c. milk, skim
- ¼ c. Parmesan cheese, grated
- 2 tbsp. corn starch

Directions:

1) Preheat oven to 350 degrees F.

2) Make the sauce by bringing milk almost to boil. Add corn starch. Constantly stir till consistency thickens.

3) Add egg yolks, cheese, nutmeg and cinnamon. Stir constantly till sauce is thick. Set aside to cool while you make the remainder.

4) Sauté beef and onion with nonstick spray. Drain.

5) Add the oregano, tomatoes and wine. Simmer for 30 minutes.

6) Place the eggplant on cookie sheet. Grill till browned lightly.

7) Add oat bran, egg whites and cheese to the meat sauce. Remove from heat.

8) Spray cooking dish with nonstick spray. Layer dish using half of eggplant, all of meat mixture and then remainder of eggplant.

9) Pour sauce over top. Add nutmeg and Parmesan cheese.

10) Place in the oven. Bake for an hour. Serve.

Sticky Asian Chicken

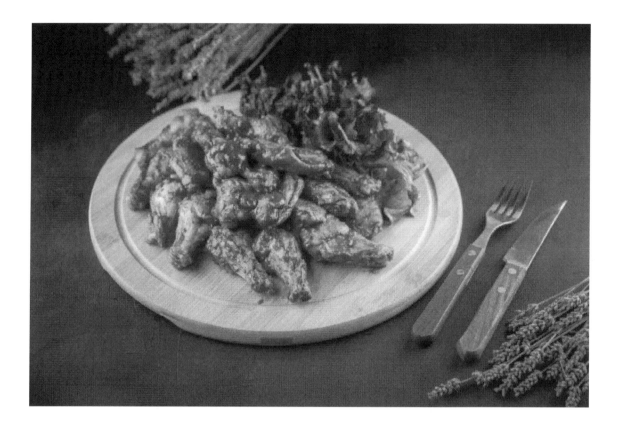

The sticky Asian Chicken boasts outstanding favors and sweet taste. The meal is tender, sticky and yummy, thus serving as a better option to start with in the morning. It will only take you less than thirty minutes to get everything done.

Servings: 3

Cook time: 25 minutes

Ingredients:

- 2 tsp. chili paste
- 8 chicken tenders, boneless and skinless
- 3 tbsp. soy sauce, low sodium
- 3 tbsp. vinegar, balsamic
- 1 tsp. Splenda

Directions:

1) Brown each side of chicken pieces in skillet pre-sprayed with non-stick spray. Thighs will usually take about five minutes per side, and tenders will often be done in three minutes per side.

2) Combine remainder of ingredients in sauce pan. Bring to boil. Simmer for five minutes. Mixture should have thickened.

3) After chicken is browned, add sauce to skillet. Cook for about five to 10 minutes for chicken thighs or five to seven minutes for chicken tenders. Serve.

Dukan Tacos

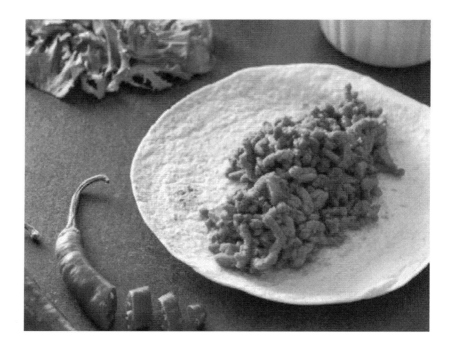

If you need to start your morning active and in a tasty manner, the Dukan Tacos should be your go-for meal. It is a healthier way to try this meal at home as it is loaded with the best ingredients that will cater to your health needs.

Servings: 4

Cook time: 15 minutes

Ingredients:

For taco shells

- ½ tsp. garlic powder
- 1 egg, large
- ½ c. cheddar cheese shreds, fat free
- ¼ c. bran, oat
- 1 scoop protein powder, unflavored
- ¼ tsp. salt, kosher
- ½ tsp. onion powder
- 2 tbsp. water, filtered
- ¼ tsp. pepper, ground

For the beef

- 2/3 c. water, filtered
- 1 packet seasoning mix, taco
- Cheddar cheese shreds, fat free
- 1 lb. ground beef, extra lean

Directions:

To create taco shells

1) Blend all ingredients outside of water in a food processor.

2) Add 1-2 tbsp. of water to create your desired consistency.

3) Preheat a pan with non-stick spray over med-high.

4) Pour 1/4 of the batter in the pan. Tilt and form a five to six-inch tortilla.

5) Cook for two or three minutes till the edge forms a crust. Flip. Cook for one to two more minutes.

To prepare meat and assemble the tacos

1) Brown beef lightly in large size pan.

2) Add taco seasoning and 2/3 cup of water. Stir and bring to boil.

3) Reduce to simmer and simmer for five minutes.

4) Serve seasoned beef and chosen condiments on homemade tortillas.

Lunch recipes

Healthy food is essential for the general growth of the body. To some extent, some play a medicinal role. In these lunch recipes, there are different meals with each playing a critical role. Some of the recipes are a perfect match for anyone experiencing busy lunch hours. During lunchtime, you might be fixed and probably won't have enough time to prepare the best meals for yourself. However, this section entails a set of meals that are easy and quick to prepare hence saving you the time you could have spent doing a task. All of them stick to the needs of the Dukan diet.

Leaf Frittata

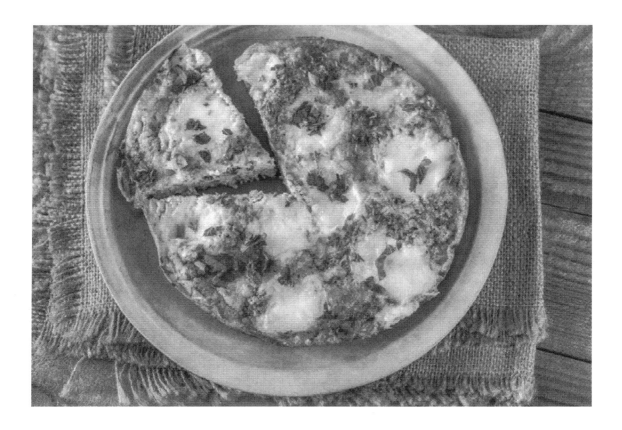

It is another frittata that requires no form of complexities while in the preparation process. In only a few minutes, your leaf frittata will be ready and good to be shared among workmates. Enjoy its tantalizing taste.

Servings: 2

Cook time: 20 minutes

Ingredients:

- ¼ tsp. salt
- ¼ tsp. dill
- 2 eggs
- ½ lb. leaf
- 1 tbsp. olive oil
- 2 oz. cheddar cheese
- ½ red onion
- 1 garlic clove

Directions

1) In a bowl, whisk eggs with salt and cheese

2) In a frying pan heat olive oil and pour egg mixture

3) Add remaining ingredients and mix well

4) Serve when ready

Vietnamese Beef

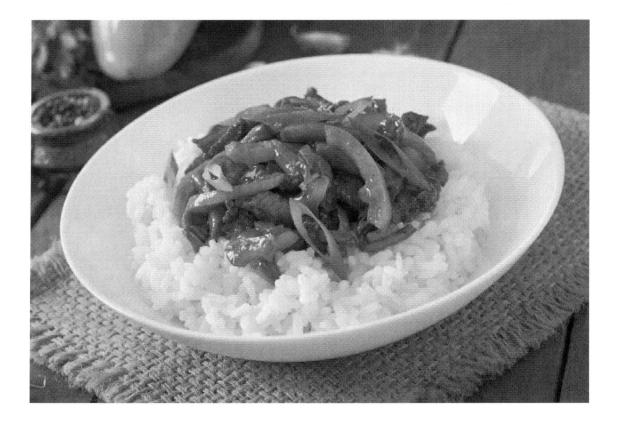

It is a go-to meal when you are approaching the lunch session. Beef can be made even sweeter with the incorporation of essential and sweet ingredients. But it can be more delicious when prepared in the Vietnamese way. Take a break for lunch and enjoy this mouth-watering delicacy.

Servings: 3

Cook time: 10 minutes

Ingredients:

- 2 tbsp. soy sauce
- 4 garlic cloves, crushed
- 10 oz. sirloin steak, sliced into ½ inch cubes
- 45g oyster sauce
- ¼ tsp. vegetable oil
- 1 tsp. minced ginger

Directions:

1) In a bowl, grate ginger. Mix in vegetable oyster sauce and soy sauce. Mix well.

2) Add beef cubes and marinate for an hour in the ref.

3) On high fire, place a nonstick skillet and heat oil. Add garlic. Then, stir fry for a minute or until lightly browned.

4) Add beef and cook on medium fire for 10 minutes or until desired doneness is reached.

5) Remove from pan and serve.

Jicama Frittata

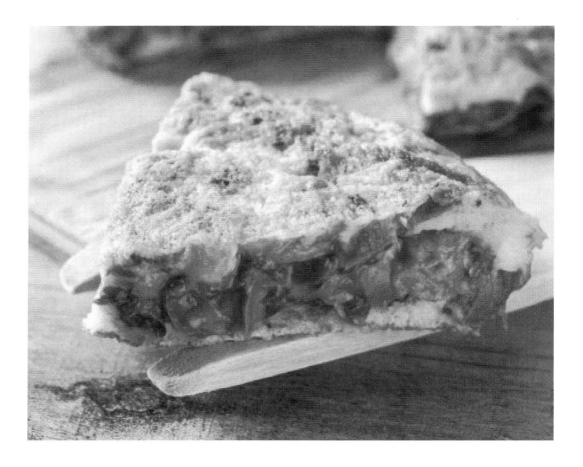

Just like any other frittata, you will enjoy the flavors of this one. Just a slight change through the incorporation of jicama and other key ingredients. You will enjoy its sweetness.

Servings: 2

Cook time: 20 minutes

Ingredients:

- ¼ tsp. dill
- 2 oz. parmesan cheese
- 1 tbsp. olive oil
- ½ red onion
- ½ c. jicama
- ¼ tsp. salt
- 2 eggs
- 1 garlic clove

Directions

1) In a bowl, whisk eggs with salt and parmesan cheese

2) In a frying pan, heat olive oil and pour the egg mixture

3) Add remaining ingredients and mix well

4) Serve when ready

Mexican Corn Dip

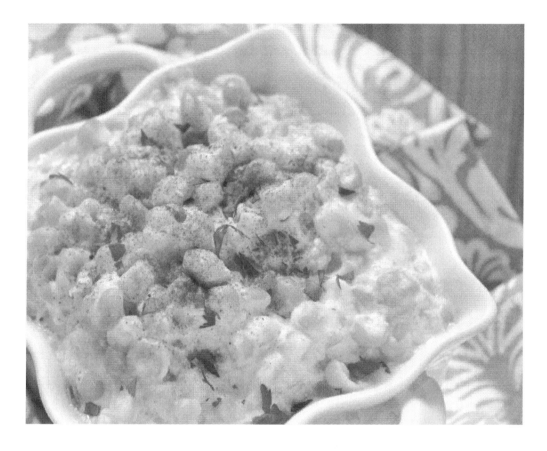

The Mexican corn dip boasts outstanding flavors that will keep you yearning for more. Make your lunch different by trying this Mexican Corn Dip.

Servings: 2

Cook time: 20 minutes

Ingredients:

- 1 jalapeno pepper
- 2 tbsp. cilantro
- 1 tbsp. butter
- 1 tbsp. lime juice
- 1 tsp. chili powder
- 2 c. kernels
- 1 red onion
- ½ c. mayonnaise

Directions

1) First, in a skillet, melt butter over medium heat

2) Add corn and cook for 5-6 minutes

3) Add chili powder, jalapeno, red onion and cook on low heat

4) Add lime juice, mayonnaise and cook for another 2-3 minutes

5) Lastly, remove from heat. Stir in cilantro and serve with tortilla chips

Seafood Spanish Style

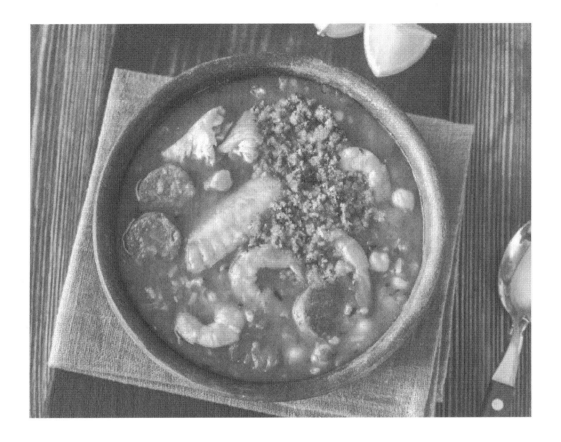

Just a few ingredients with an already prepared seafood mix can serve anyone perfectly as a substitute for lunch. The meal is delicious, and your friends will love it too. A single try will make you yearn to prepare it more.

Servings: 2

Cook time: 10 minutes

Ingredients:

- 1 garlic clove, minced
- ½ red chili, minced
- 1 packet chilled pre-cooked seafood mix
- Pepper and salt
- 1 tsp. tomato puree

Directions:

1) On medium high fire, place a medium nonstick fry pan and grease with cooking spray.

2) Once heated, add garlic and sauté for 2 to 3 minutes or until lightly browned.

3) Add seafood mix, cover and cook for 5 minutes or until water has evaporated fully.

4) Add tomato puree and mix well.

5) Season with pepper and salt to taste. Toss to mix well.

6) Cook for another minute.

7) Remove from pan. Then, transfer to a serving plate, serve and enjoy.

Simple Pizza Recipe

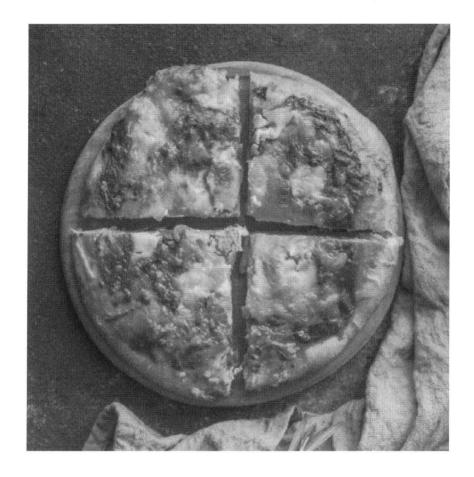

Pizza is among the most loved best foods. However, there are different versions of pizzas, and each comes with a different way of preparation. The simple pizza, as the name suggests, requires no more complex steps to get it to the table for lunch. With toppings and other essential ingredients, you can be sure to enjoy the unique taste of the simply prepared pizza.

Servings: 8

Cook time: 15 minutes

Ingredients:

- 1 c. pepperoni slices
- 1 c. olives
- 1 pizza crust
- ¼ black pepper
- ½ c. tomato sauce
- 1 c. mozzarella cheese

Directions

1) Spread tomato sauce on the pizza crust

2) Place all the toppings on the pizza crust

3) Bake the pizza at 425 F for 12-15 minutes

4) When ready remove pizza from the oven and serve

Grilled Cod

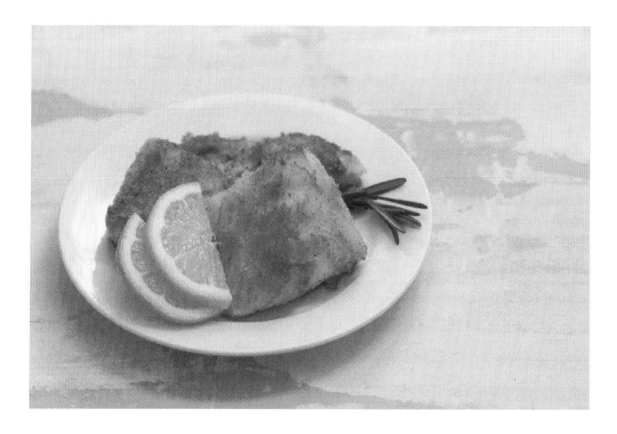

You can always make your lunch a perfect match for anyone when you prepare the grilled cod. It requires no complex steps, and therefore, you can be sure of preparing the perfect meal within a short period of time. The grilled cod is a good meal to enjoy with friends.

Servings: 3

Cook time: 18 minutes

Ingredients:

- ½ tsp. lemon pepper
- 1 tbsp. Cajun seasoning
- 2 tbsp. chopped green onions, white part only
- 1 lemon, juiced
- ¼ tsp. salt
- ¼ tsp. ground black pepper
- 2 fillets cod, halved

Directions:

1) Prepare grill by preheating to medium high for around ten minutes. Grease grate with cooking spray.

2) Meanwhile, season cod fillets (front and back) with black pepper, salt, lemon pepper and Cajun seasoning.

3) Place on hot grill. Then, cook for 3 minutes per side or until cod flakes easily. Ensure that you turn cod only once or else it may break into pieces.

4) Remove from grill, transfer to a serving plate and let it sit for 5 minutes.

5) Serve and enjoy.

Baked Mussels

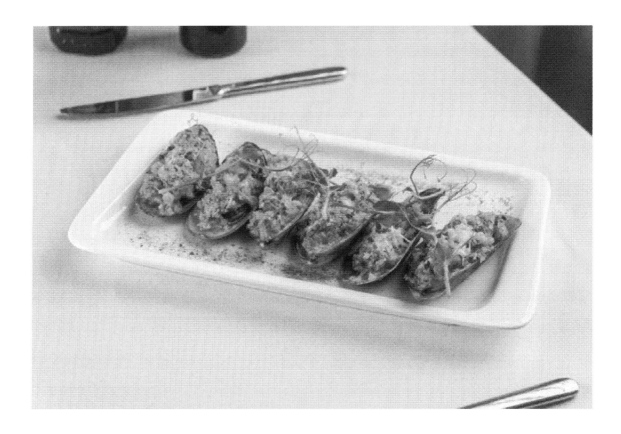

You would get outstanding tastes from trying the baked mussels. Along with other essential ingredients, you can be sure to enjoy your lunch without stress.

Servings: 2

Cook time: 25 minutes

Ingredients:

- 1-inch long ginger, peeled
- ¼ c. green onions, minced
- 3 garlic cloves, minced
- 1 lb. mussels
- 1 c. less fat cream cheese

Directions:

1) In a bowl, mix cream cheese and green onions well. Set aside.

2) In a heavy bottomed pot placed on medium high fire, add mussels, garlic and ginger.

3) Cover. Then, cook for 8 to 10 minutes or until most of the mussels have opened fully.

4) Turn off fire, uncover pot and let it cool for ten minutes.

5) One by one, remove the mussels and break off the empty shell and discard. Arrange shell with mussel on a baking sheet.

6) Meanwhile preheat the oven to 350oF.

7) Once all mussels are on the baking sheet, place cream cheese mixture on top of mussels. Ensure that you evenly place cream cheese mixture on each mussel and cover it with the cream cheese mixture well.

8) Pop mussels in the oven and bake for 10 to 15 minutes or until cream cheese are melted and bubbly.

9) Remove from oven. Then, let it rest for 5 minutes before serving.

Baked Salmon

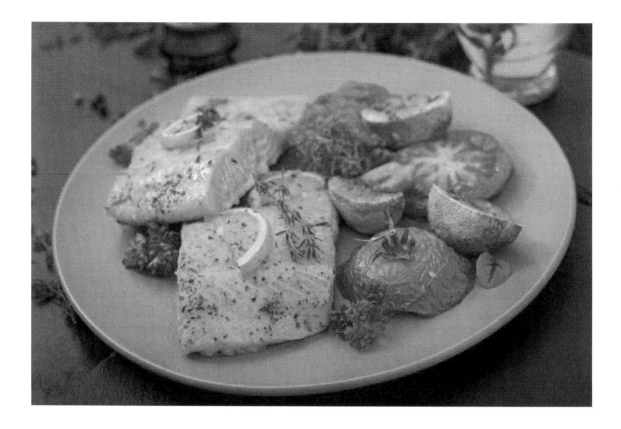

Salmon will turn your lunch session into activeness. The lunch is made even sweeter when the Salmon is baked along with other essential ingredients and spices. With it, you will stay satisfied with the whole lunch session.

Servings: 3

Cook time: 15 minutes

Ingredients:

- 1 salmon fillet
- Freshly ground black pepper
- 1 tbsp. lemon juice
- Salt

Directions:

1) In a safe oven dish, grease with cooking spray and place salmon.

2) Rub freshly ground pepper, salt and lemon juice on salmon.

3) Pop in a preheated 350oF oven. Cook for 15 minutes or until the middle of salmon is flaky.

4) Serve and enjoy.

Turkey Burger Cajun Style

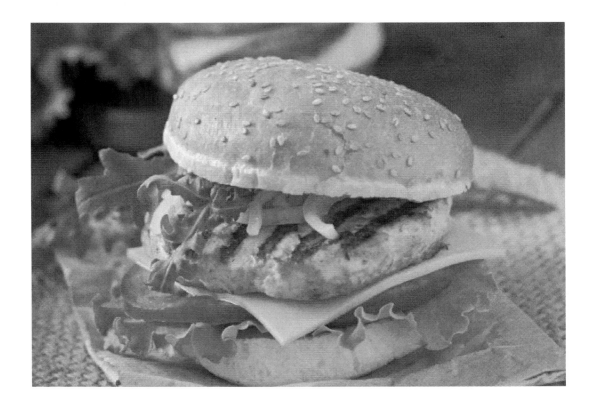

The Turkey Burger Cajun style is yet another great recipe that will make your lunch a perfect session. It entails the essential ingredients with a unique style of preparation. It does not take much time to get your meal ready.

Servings: 3

Cook time: 10 minutes

Ingredients:

- 1 tbsp. mustard
- 1 tbsp. ketchup
- 1 egg
- 1 green chili, chopped
- 2 tbsp. oat bran
- 2 garlic cloves, chopped
- 1 ½ lb. lean turkey, minced
- 1 tbsp. Cajun spice mix

Directions:

1) In a big bowl, mix garlic, chili (if using), Cajun spice mix, and egg. Whisk well together for a minute.

2) Add minced turkey and mix with hands for a minute or two.

3) Add oat bran and mix again.

4) Shape into eight small burger patties.

5) Meanwhile, on medium fire, heat a medium nonstick frying pan greased with cooking spray.

6) Once heated, add patties and cook for 3 to 5 minutes per side.

7) Remove from pan and transfer to a serving plate.

8) Serve with a side of mustard and ketchup if desired.

Zucchini Pizza

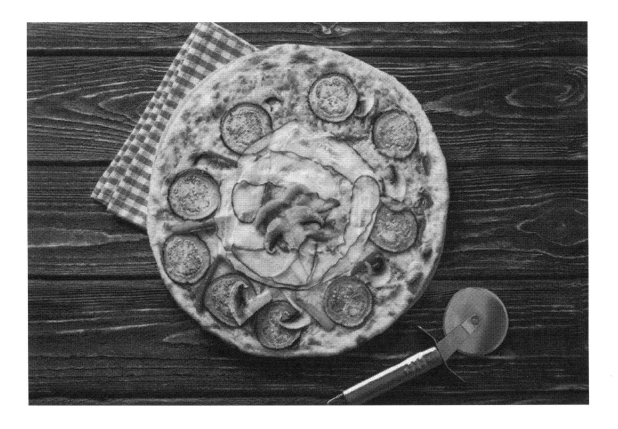

There is real greatness that comes with the preparation of zucchini pizza. Well, the normal pizza is loaded with better tastes, but the zucchini one is good enough to make your lunch session memorable. Enjoy the cheesy touch along with flavors from other ingredients.

Servings: 8

Cook time: 15 minutes

Ingredients:

- 1 c. mozzarella cheese
- 1 c. zucchini slices
- 1 c. olives
- ½ c. tomato sauce
- 1 pizza crust
- ¼ black pepper

Directions

1) Spread tomato sauce on the pizza crust

2) Place all the toppings on the pizza crust

3) Bake the pizza at 425 F for 12-15 minutes

4) When ready, remove pizza from the oven. Serve

Onion Frittata

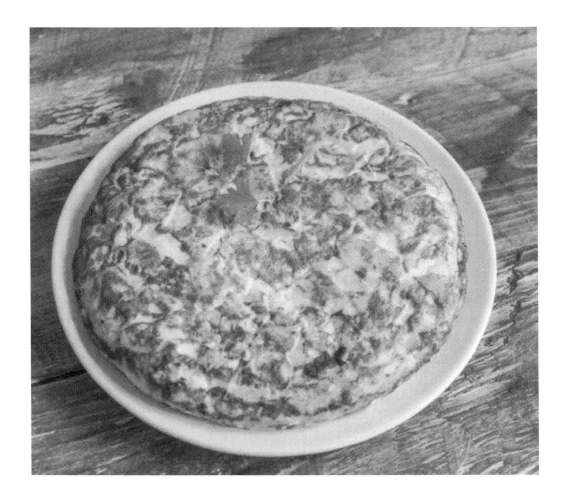

The onion frittata is prepared in a quick and simple way. You will only need two eggs, some red onion and other essential ingredients. It is a perfect fit for your lunch especially after a busy session of focusing on your work.

Servings: 2

Cook time: 20 minutes

Ingredients:

- 2 oz. cheddar cheese
- ¼ tsp. dill
- ½ red onion
- ¼ tsp. salt
- 1 tbsp. olive oil
- 2 eggs
- 1 garlic clove

Directions

1) In a bowl, whisk eggs with salt and cheese

2) In a frying pan, heat olive oil and pour the egg mixture

3) Add remaining ingredients and mix well

4) Serve when ready

Kale Frittata

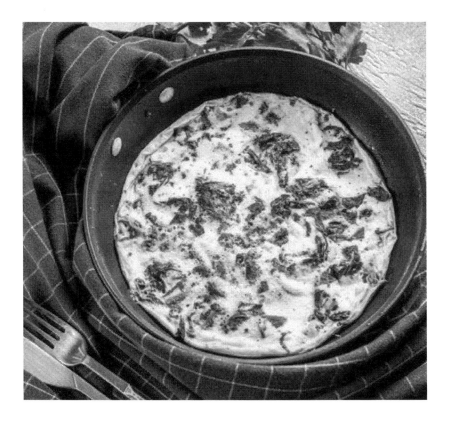

If you need to get some moment of enjoyment after busy hours of working, you can consider a meal that can energize and freshen your mind. The kale frittata is loaded with a range of nutritional roles, and with it, you can be sure to observe a healthy schedule.

Servings: 2

Cook time: 20 minutes

Ingredients:

- 2 oz. cheddar cheese
- 2 eggs
- ¼ tsp. dill
- 1 garlic clove
- 1 c. kale
- ½ red onion
- ¼ tsp. salt
- 1 tbsp. olive oil

Directions

1) In a skillet, sauté kale until tender

2) In a bowl, whisk eggs with salt and cheese

3) In a frying pan, heat olive oil and pour egg mixture

4) Add remaining ingredients and mix well

5) When ready, serve with sautéed kale

Broccoli Frittata

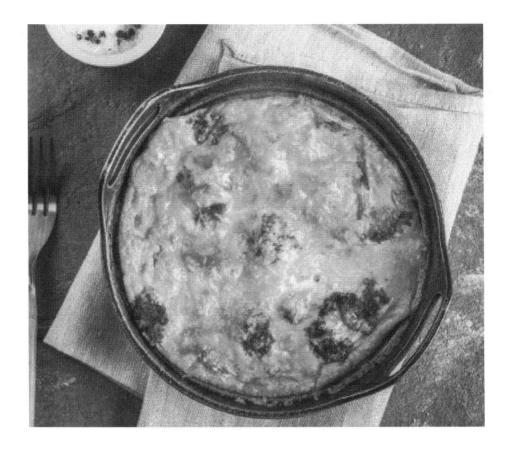

Among the most excellent ways to get your lunch sessions to work well for you is to try the broccoli frittata. The meal is quick and easy to prepare, and therefore, you will have no stress waiting for hours and hours.

Servings: 2

Cook time: 20 minutes

Ingredients:

- ½ red onion
- 1 garlic clove
- 2 eggs
- ¼ tsp. salt
- 1 tbsp. olive oil
- 2 oz. cheddar cheese
- 1 c. broccoli
- ¼ tsp. dill

Directions

1) In a skillet, sauté broccoli until tender

2) In a bowl, whisk eggs with salt and cheese

3) In a frying pan, heat olive oil and pour the egg mixture

4) Add remaining ingredients and mix well

5) When ready, serve with sautéed broccoli

Cauliflower Sandwich

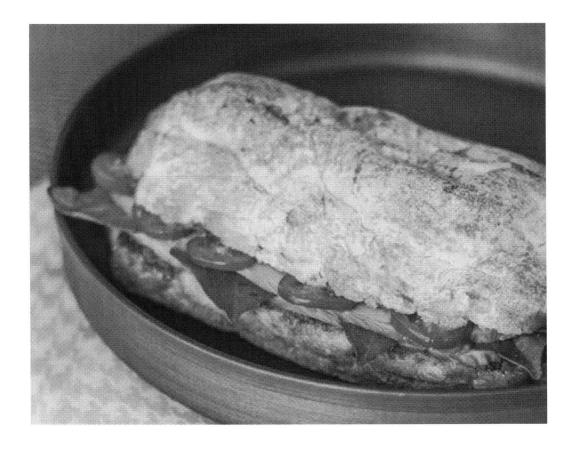

This cauliflower sandwich constitutes a set of ingredients that are essential for your child's body health as well as your health. It is a sweet delicacy that you should not afford to miss.

Servings: 2

Cook time: 30 minutes

Ingredients:

- 1 garlic clove
- ½ red onion
- 4 slices gluten-free bread
- 1 head cauliflower
- 1 avocado
- 4 tbsp. olive oil
- ¼ tsp. salt
- 2 tbsp. tahini

Directions

1) Toss the cauliflower with olive oil. Then, roast at 400 F for 22-25 minutes

2) In a saucepan, sauté the onion until soft

3) Add roasted cauliflower, tahini, olive oil, salt and cook for 1-2 minutes

4) Place everything in a blender. Then, blend until smooth

5) Spread mixture over bread slices

6) Serve when ready

Avocado Boats

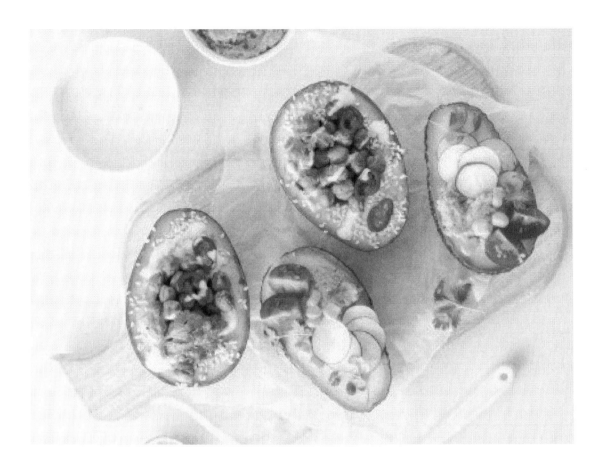

Avocado boats are some of the simplest meals you can opt for during the lunch period. The meal is vital for body growth as it is loaded with the essential ingredients you will need. It is tasty and enjoyable.

Servings: 2

Cook time: 10 minutes

Ingredients:

- ½ c. tahini
- ¼ red onion
- 2 avocados
- 1 can chickpeas
- 1 tbsp. dill
- ½ tsp. garlic powder
- 1 tbsp. mustard
- ¼ tsp. turmeric

Directions

1) Cut avocado in half and scoop out part of the interior

2) In a bowl, combine together chickpeas with onion, turmeric, dill, garlic, tahini and mustard

3) Mix well and spoon mixture into avocado halves

4) Serve when ready

Leek Quiche

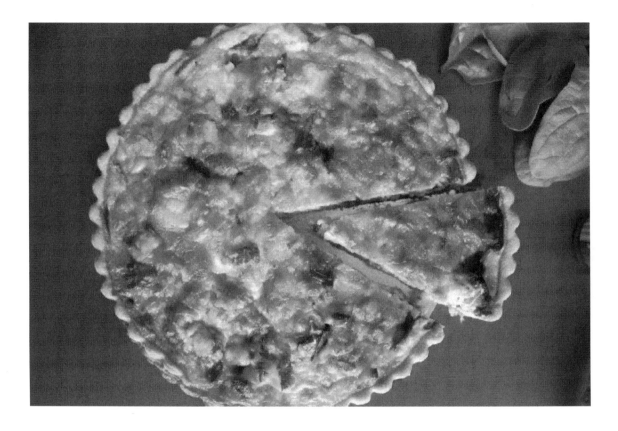

If you need a perfect taste of quiche, then you can try Leek Quiche. It is a perfect choice of meal to serve for lunch. You can enjoy it along with friends and other workmates.

Servings: 4

Cook time: 50 minutes

Ingredients:

- 1 pie crust
- ½ c. vanilla yogurt
- 1 c. almond milk
- 1 bunch asparagus
- 1 leek
- ¼ tsp. salt
- 2 eggs
- 1 tbsp. butter

Directions

1) In a saucepan, melt butter, add leek, asparagus, pepper, and salt, and cook until vegetables are soft

2) In a bowl, combine eggs, milk, yogurt and mix well

3) Place egg mixture on the pie crust

4) Top with asparagus and leek

5) Bake at 375 F for 40-45 minutes

6) When ready, remove from the oven. Serve

Brussels Sprout Salad

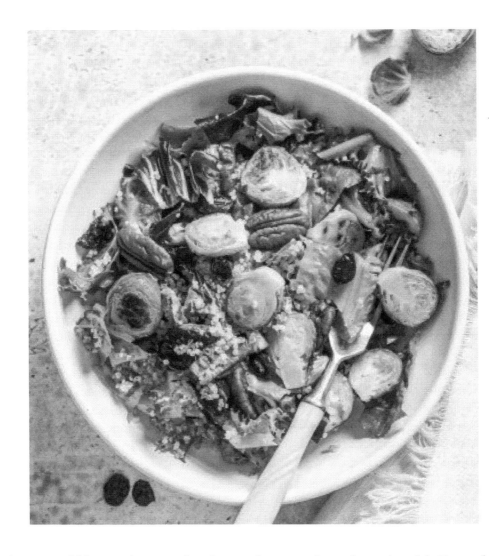

It is also a good idea to give your lunch a perfect experience by trying this Brussels sprout salad. It won't take you much time, and, therefore, no need to getting worried about how long it will take to get it done.

Servings: 2

Cook time: 5 minutes

Ingredients:

- 1 tbsp. olive oil
- Herbs
- ½ c. celery
- 1 garlic clove
- 1 c. shallots
- 8 Brussels sprouts
- 1 tbsp. thyme leaves

Directions

1) In a bowl, mix all ingredients and mix well

2) Serve with dressing

Cobb Salad

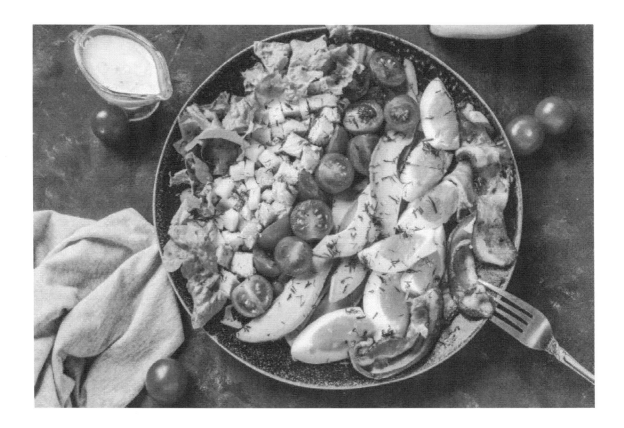

A salad like Cobb salad can always be a perfect match for your lunch as it is loaded with a set of substantial ingredients. You will enjoy its taste along with flavors from other ingredients.

Servings: 2

Cook time: 5 minutes

Ingredients:

- 1 tbsp. lemon juice
- ¼ tsp. pistachios
- ¼ c. mint leaves
- 1 c. cooked quinoa
- 1 bunch scallions
- 1 c. tomatoes
- ¼ c. olive oil
- 1 avocado

Directions

1) In a bowl, mix all ingredients and mix well

2) Serve with dressing

Ice Salad

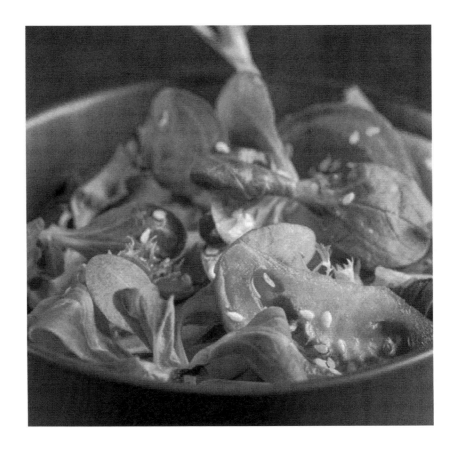

With turnips, radishes, beets, walnuts, carrots and other essential ingredients incorporated together, you are sure of this salad that is healthy for your body. Enjoy it.

Servings: 2

Cook time: 5 minutes

Ingredients:

- ¼ lb. turnips
- 4 oz. Parmesan
- ¼ lb. radishes
- ¼ lb. carrots
- 1 c. walnuts
- ¼ lb. fennel
- ¼ lb. beets
- 2 garlic cloves

Directions

1) In a bowl, mix all ingredients and mix well

2) Serve with dressing

Endive & Fig Salad

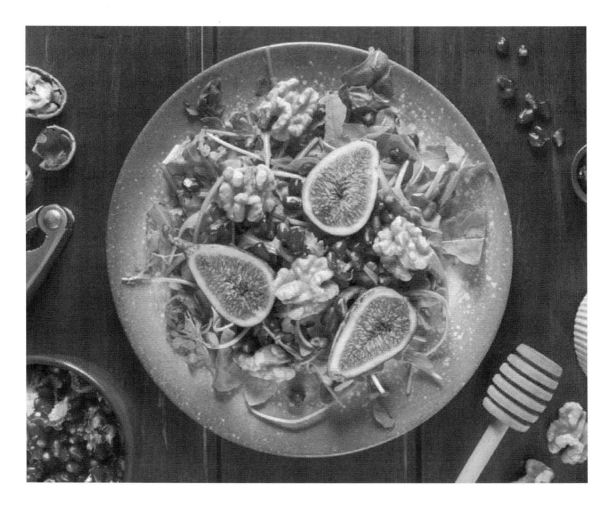

This endive and fig salad is nutritious and serves as a better meal for your lunch. The preparation doesn't take much time. Therefore, with a busy afternoon, you can be sure that the salad is a perfect match.

Servings: 2

Cook time: 5 minutes

Ingredients:

- 4 endives
- ¼ c. black olives
- 2 tbsp. lemon juice
- 1 c. watermelon
- 1 tbsp. honey
- 10 oz. figs

Directions

1) In a bowl, mix all ingredients and mix well

2) Serve with dressing

Bacon Salad

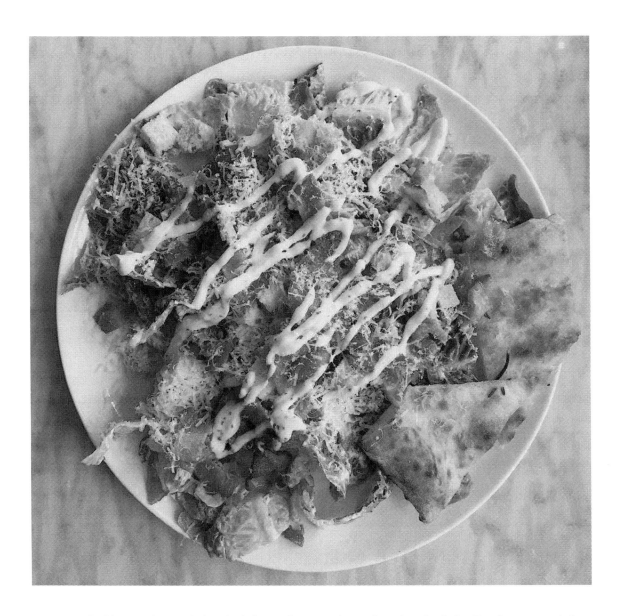

Bacon salad is another quick salad that suits your busy lunch schedule. Furthermore, it has a range of ingredients that are a good match for anyone whose major aim is to observe a healthy lunch schedule. Enjoy the outstanding taste.

Servings: 2

Cook time: 5 minutes

Ingredients:

- 2 romaine hearts
- 1 lb. tomatoes
- ¼ c. mayonnaise
- ½ bunch chives
- 2 tbsp. lemon juice
- 7 bacon slices
- 1 avocado

Directions

1) In a bowl, mix all ingredients and mix well

2) Serve with dressing

Kabocha Salad

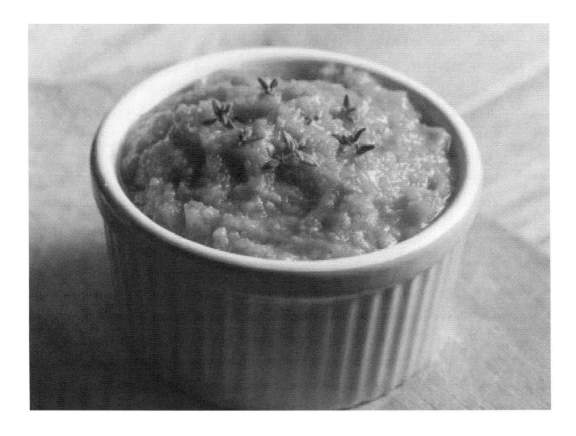

In just a few minutes, your Kabocha salad will be ready. The salad is loaded with a range of few ingredients that are quite vital for body health. You will enjoy it.

Servings: 2

Cook time: 5 minutes

Ingredients:

- 2 tbsp. butter
- 2 tbsp. balsamic vinegar
- 2 kabochas
- 2 tbsp. lemon juice
- 64 oz. Brussels sprouts
- 2 tbsp. olive oil
- 1 garlic clove

Directions

1) In a bowl, mix all ingredients and mix well

2) Serve with dressing

Watermelon Salad

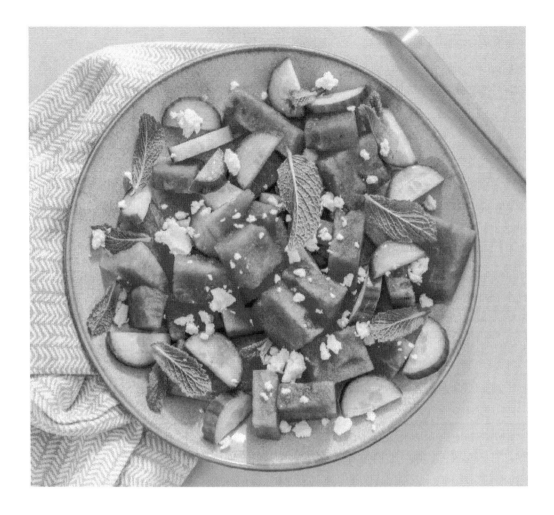

Enjoy the favor of watermelon along with other ingredients through this salad. Just like other salads, it will not take you more time. Try it and enjoy it.

Servings: 2

Cook time: 5 minutes

Ingredients:

- ½ c. peanuts
- ¼ c. almonds
- 2 lb. watermelon
- 3 sprigs basil
- 1 tbsp. lemon juice
- ½ c. walnuts

Directions

1) In a bowl, mix all ingredients and mix well

2) Serve with dressing

Dinner Recipes

Your dinner needs to be unique especially after experiencing a long and tiresome day. You need to treat yourself to at least a special meal. In this section, dinner recipes have been specially chosen to ensure that you have a nice and easier time preparing them. Most of the recipes have easily affordable and accessible ingredients and, therefore, no need for straining. The recipes also adhere to the rules of the Dukan diet. Try preparing the meals, and you will have more fantastic dinner sessions.

Grilled Lamb Chops

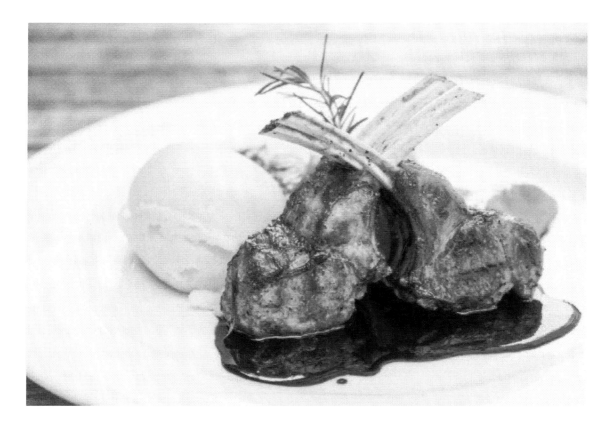

Your dinner cannot be close to perfect without a taste of lamb chops. It is even sweeter when the lamb chops are grilled with other essential ingredients incorporated.

Servings: 3

Cook time: 1 hour 6 minutes

Ingredients:

- ½ tsp. black pepper
- ¼ c. distilled white vinegar
- 2 lb. lamb chops
- 1 tbsp. garlic minced
- 1 onion, sliced thinly
- 2 tsp. salt

Directions:

1) In a re-sealable bag, mix onion, garlic, pepper, salt and vinegar. Seal the bag and shake until salt is dissolved.

2) Add lamb chops into the bag and marinate in the ref for at least two hours. While ensuring that you turn bag after an hour to ensure that all sides are marinated well.

3) On medium high fire, preheat grill and grease grate with cooking spray.

4) Remove lamb chops from bag and cover bony ends with foil. Place on the grate and grill for at least 3 minutes per side or until desired doneness is reached.

5) Remove from grill, transfer to plate, serve and enjoy.

Dijon-Worcestershire Marinated Grilled Flank Steak

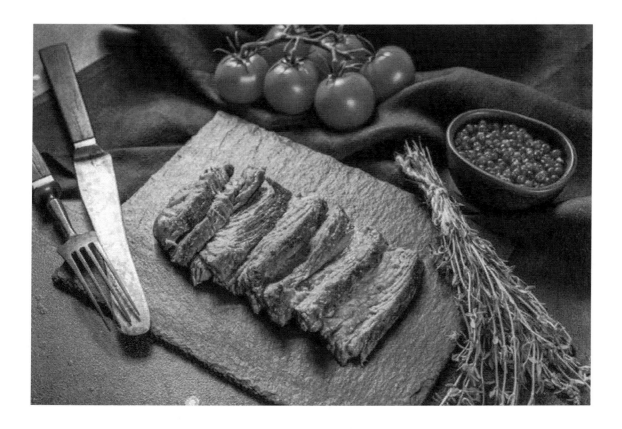

For a highly valued and sweet meal that can add delightful moments to your dinner routine, this meal is a perfect option. Give it a try, and be sure to enjoy it.

Servings: 6

Cook time: 10 minutes

Ingredients:

- 2 tbsp. fresh lemon juice
- ½ c. vegetable oil
- 1/3 c. soy sauce
- ½ tsp. ground black pepper
- 2 garlic cloves, minced
- 1 ½ tbsp. Worcestershire sauce
- 1 ½ lb. flank steak
- 1 tbsp. Dijon mustard
- ¼ c. red wine vinegar

Directions:

1) Thoroughly mix ground black pepper, garlic, mustard, Worcestershire sauce, lemon juice, vinegar, soy sauce, and oil in a medium bowl.

2) Place steak in a shallow glass dish. Then, pour the marinade over it. Turn meat to coat with the marinade, refrigerate for 6 hours and turn to coat meat every hour.

3) Grease grate, and on medium-high fire, preheat.

4) Grill meat for 5 minutes per side, and cook to desired doneness.

5) Serve and enjoy!

Mushroom, Beans, and Carrots Stir Fry

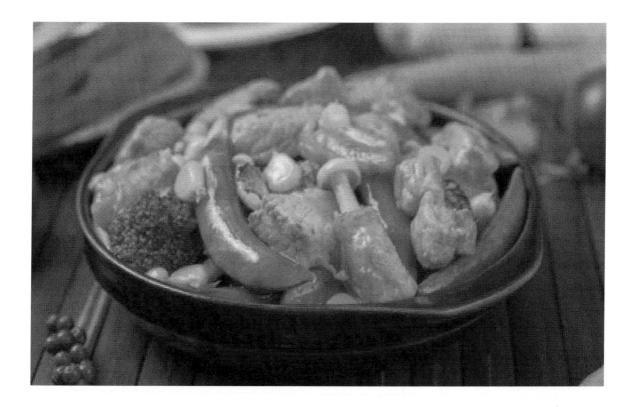

A more convenient way of incorporating veggies into your normal dinner routine is to try this type of recipe. It is a perfect match for you, especially when you are busy. Therefore, not much time is taken in getting everything of the recipe done.

Servings: 4

Cook time: 15 minutes

Ingredients:

- 1 ½ c. fresh mushrooms
- 4 carrots, julienned
- 2 tbsp. butter
- 1 tsp. salt
- ½ tsp. dried thyme
- ½ lb. green beans cut into 2-inch pieces

Directions:

1) On medium-high heat, place a medium saucepan, and heat butter.

2) Add mushrooms, green beans, carrots, thyme, and salt.

3) Stir-fry until beans are crisp tender, around 15 minutes.

4) Remove from fire, transfer to a serving plate, serve and enjoy.

Beef Kebabs

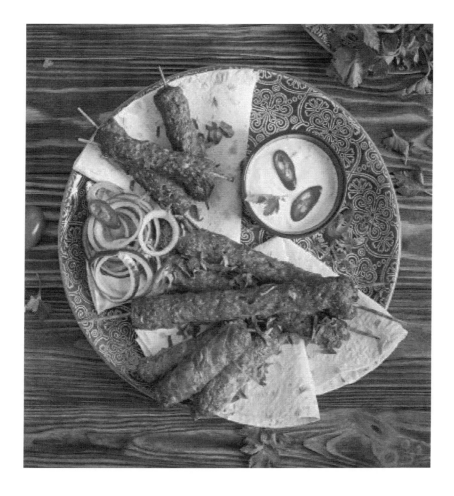

Another way of giving your family members a memorable treat is to try these beef kebabs. They are sweet and delicious.

Servings: 3

Cook time: 10 minutes

Ingredients:

- ¼ c. fresh lemon juice
- 1 tbsp. cider vinegar
- ¼ tsp. thyme
- 14 oz. beef fillet
- 1 bay leaf
- 2 tbsp. Dijon mustard
- ¼ c. low sodium soy sauce

Directions:

1) Cut beef into 1-inch cubes.

2) In a bowl, mix the remaining ingredients thoroughly.

3) Add meat to seasoning mixture and marinade for at least two hours inside the ref. Ensure that you flip meat after an hour to marinate all sides of the meat.

4) Skewer the beef in Barbecue sticks and discard marinade.

5) Place kebabs in preheated grill on medium high fire and grill for 3 to 5 minutes per se or until desired doneness.

6) Remove from grill. Then, let it rest for 5 minutes before serving.

Sautéed Veggies in Garlic Oil

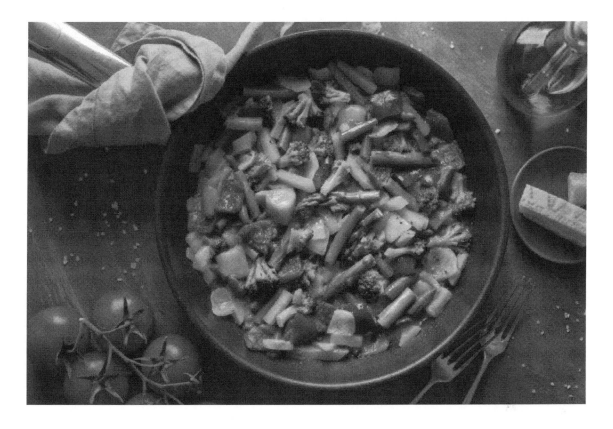

As a way of maintaining the Dukan diet, these sautéed veggies in garlic oil will give you a healthy start during your dinner. Enjoy it with family members.

Servings: 4

Cook time: 5 minutes

Ingredients:

- 1 lb. asparagus ends trimmed
- 1 lb. carrots, halved lengthwise
- Ground pepper
- 2 tbsp. garlic oil
- Coarse salt

Directions:

1) In a pan of simmering water, place asparagus and carrots in a steamer basket and steam while covered for 5 minutes or until tender.

2) Place cooked carrots and asparagus on a serving plate and garnish with chopped cloves; season with pepper and salt and drizzle with garlic oil.

3) Serve and enjoy!

Chicken Curry

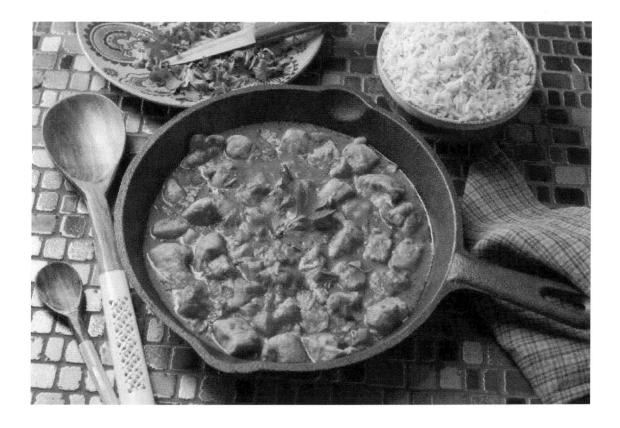

This chicken curry is made sweeter and hotter with the addition of some cayenne pepper and cinnamon. It requires a variety of ingredients to achieve the desired outcome. Therefore, you are sure to enjoy it from a range of minerals.

Servings: 3

Cook time: 28 minutes

Ingredients:

- 1 tsp. ground cinnamon
- ½ tsp. cayenne pepper
- ½ lemon, juiced
- 1 tsp. paprika
- 1 tomato, sliced into wedges
- 3 tbsp. curry powder
- 1 small onion, chopped
- 2 skinless, boneless chicken breast halves, cut into ½-inch cubes
- 3 tbsp. olive oil
- 2 garlic cloves, minced
- Salt.
- ½ tsp. truvia
- ½ tsp. grated fresh ginger
- ½ c. water
- 1 bay leaf
- 1 c. zero fat yogurt

Directions:

1) In a large nonstick saucepan greased with cooking spray on medium high fire, add onion and tomatoes.

2) Stir fry for 4 minutes or until lightly wilted. Add salt, truvia, ginger, bay leaf, paprika, cinnamon, curry powder and garlic. Stir fry for 2 minutes.

3) Add chicken breasts and stir fry for 5 minutes.

4) Add ½ cup of water, cover and cook for another 15 to 20 minutes.

5) Add yogurt, cook until heated through.

6) Remove from pan, serve and enjoy.

Salad Made of Winter Greens

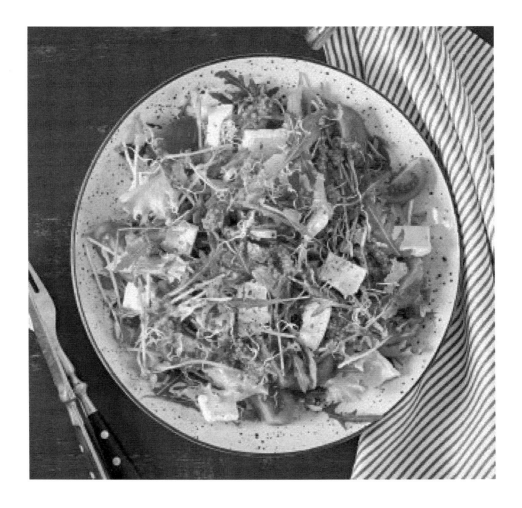

If you need a fresh, sweet and nutritious salad made with garden ingredients, you can try this recipe. Enjoy its fruity and tasty touch.

Servings: 4

Cook time: 10 minutes

Ingredients:

- 1 tbsp. oregano, crushed
- 1 Bosc pear, cubed
- ¼ freshly crushed peppercorns
- ½ tsp. salt
- 1 tsp. Dijon mustard
- 1 ½ tsp. chili powder
- ¼ small head red cabbage, chopped
- 1 garlic clove, minced
- 4 collard leaves, trimmed and finely chopped
- 1 tbsp. wildflower honey
- 3 tbsp. balsamic vinegar
- 1 head romaine lettuce, chopped
- 2 tbsp. raisins
- 6 tbsp. olive oil
- 1/3 bunch kale, trimmed and chopped
- 7 walnut halves crushed
- ½ orange bell pepper, diced
- 5 cherry tomatoes, halved
- ½ carrot grated
- ½ Florida avocado, peeled, pitted and diced
- ½ Bermuda onion, finely diced
- ½ orange bell pepper, diced

Directions:

1) In a large bowl, mix raisins, walnuts, tomatoes, carrot, avocado, orange bell pepper, onion, pear, cabbage, romaine, kale, and collard greens.

2) Over a medium bowl, combine black pepper, salt, garlic, mustard, chili powder, oregano, honey, vinegar, and olive oil in a lidded jar. Close the jar and vigorously shake concoction; pour over a large bowl of salad greens.

3) Toss to mix.

4) Serve, and enjoy!

Meat Loaf

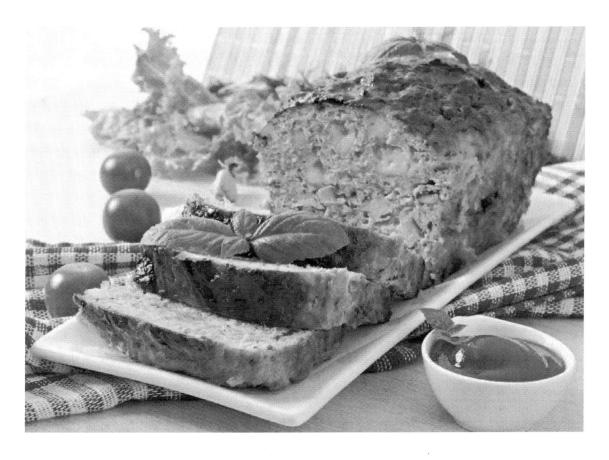

This meatloaf is tasty and sweet. It entails a variety of ingredients that are quite vital for your body's health.

Servings: 4

Cook time: 35 minutes

Ingredients:

- 1 ½ lb. ground beef
- 1 tbsp. garlic salt
- 2 ½ tbsp. chili powder
- 1 tbsp. garlic pepper seasoning
- 1 tbsp. Worcestershire sauce
- 2 eggs

Directions:

1) Preheat oven to 375oF and grease a loaf pan with cooking spray.

2) Mix eggs, Worcestershire sauce and ground beef in a large bowl.

3) Season with garlic pepper, garlic salt, and chili powder. Mix well again.

4) Place mixture into greased loaf pan. Then, press to form a loaf.

5) Pop in the oven. Then, bake for 35 minutes.

6) Remove from oven. Let it stand for minutes before serving and slicing.

Tofu Stir Fry

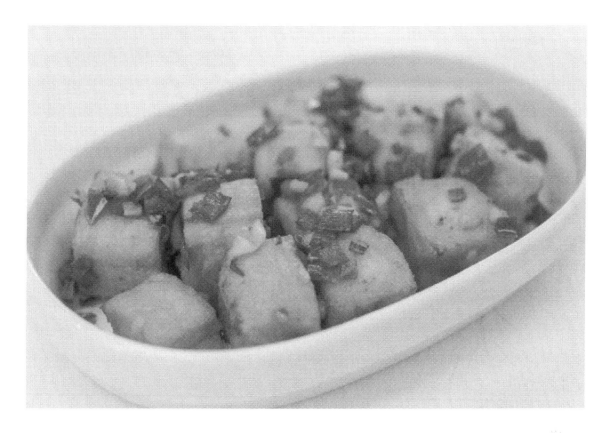

Just a few ingredients are required in the preparation process of the tofu. In about half an hour, your tofu will be ready.

Servings: 3

Cook time: 32 minutes

Ingredients:

- 2 tsp. minced garlic
- 1 tbsp. tamari
- 2 lb. firm tofu
- 1 lime
- 2 tsp. minced fresh ginger root

Directions:

1) On medium high fire, place a medium nonstick saucepan and grease with cooking spray.

2) Stir fry ginger and garlic for two minutes.

3) Add tamari and tofu. Stir to mix.

4) Cover pan and lower fire to medium and cook for 20 to 30 minutes while ensuring to stir every 5 minutes.

5) Remove from pan. Then, transfer to a serving bowl.

6) Squeeze lime juice on top and serve.

Squash, Zucchini, and Eggplant Garlic Scramble

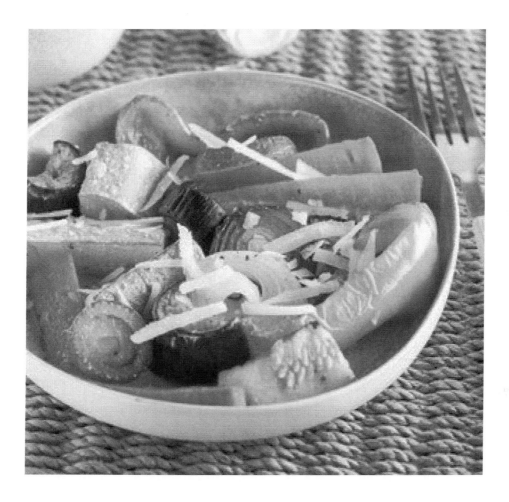

Enjoy the garlicky taste along with other spices. The scramble is healthier as it includes the best ingredients that will take care of your health.

Servings: 4

Cook time: 10 minutes

Ingredients:

- ½ lb. zucchini, sliced into edible pieces
- ½ lb. yellow squash, sliced into edible pieces
- 3 tbsp. oyster sauce
- 1 onion, sliced into ½ inch wide strips
- ½ lb. eggplant, sliced into edible pieces
- 2 tbsp. finely minced garlic
- ¼ tsp. salt
- 2 tbsp. peanut oil

Directions:

1) Over medium-high heat, place a large saucepan and heat oil for 2 minutes.

2) Add onions and garlic. Then, stir fry for half a minute.

3) Add all vegetables, and fry. Add salt, and continue stir-frying for 4-5 minutes.

4) Once veggies have started to soften, add oyster sauce.

5) Cook for another two minutes, stirring periodically.

6) Transfer to a serving plate. Enjoy it while hot.

Garlic-Braised Garden Greens

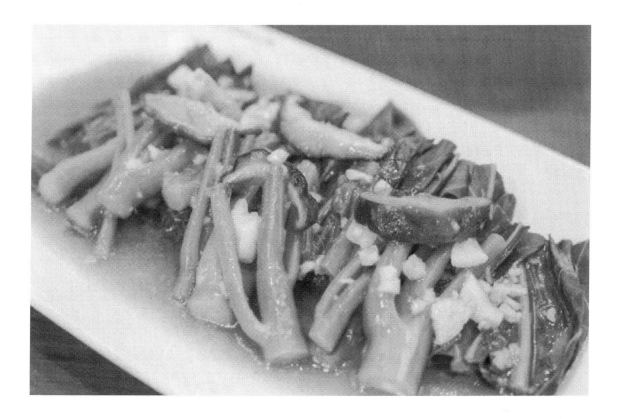

Among the crucial elements of this recipe are collard, mustard and kale greens. Incorporation of other ingredients adds a constructive, healthy role and makes the meal sweeter.

Servings: 1

Cook time: 1 minute

Ingredients:

- 4 oz. greens
- ¼ tsp. red pepper flakes
- 1/8 tsp. sea salt
- 1 garlic cloves

Directions:

1) On medium-high fire, place a large skillet and heat oil.

2) Add garlic, and sauté until golden brown.

3) Add greens, and continue sautéing until nearly wilted.

4) Add pepper flakes and salt while continuing to stir.

5) Cook for a minute more. Then, remove from fire and serve.

Lemon Poppy and Fruits on Garden Salad

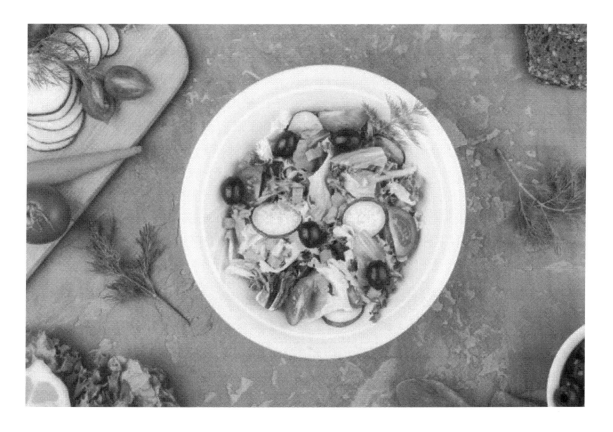

Enjoy the texture and touch of this garden salad. It is delicious, sweet and mouthwatering.

Servings: 12

Cook time: 15 minutes

Ingredients:

- ½ c. white sugar
- ½ c. lemon juice
- 1 pear peeled, cored and diced
- 1 c. cashews
- 1 tbsp. poppy seeds
- 2/3 c. vegetable oil
- 1 apple peeled, cored and diced
- 4 oz. shredded Swiss cheese
- 1 head romaine lettuce, torn into smaller pieces
- ½ tsp. salt
- 1 tsp. Dijon style prepared mustard
- 2 tsp. diced onion

Directions:

1) Blend salt, mustard, onion, lemon juice, and sugar in a food processor until smooth.

2) Slowly pour in oil while continuing to blend at low speed until thick and creamy.

3) Add lemon poppy seeds, and pulse for a second or two.

4) Combine pear, apple, cashews, cheese, and lettuce in a big salad bowl.

5) Pour in dressing, and toss to mix.

6) Serve, and enjoy!

Simply Grilled Asparagus

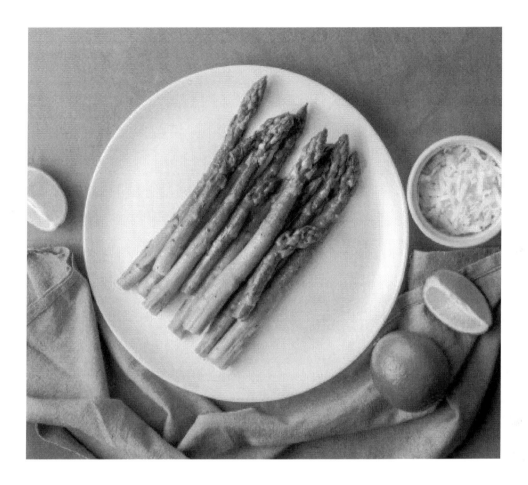

This meal is loaded with many ingredients, and among the major ones is asparagus. Usually, asparagus is a great source of vitamin K and, therefore, critical for any individual suffering from unique kinds of diseases. You can try the recipe since it also serves medicinal roles.

Servings: 4

Cook time: 10 minutes

Ingredients:

- 3 tbsp. extra virgin olive oil
- 1 lb. asparagus
- 1 lemon
- Black ground pepper
- Kosher salt

Directions:

1) In a container, place asparagus, and season with pepper, salt, and 2 tbsp olive oil. Toss to coat.

2) On a preheated grill and oiled grate, grill asparagus around 5-8 minutes, or until tender.

3) Transfer to a serving plate, drizzle with remaining olive oil and garnish with lemon if desired.

Fresh Garden Salad

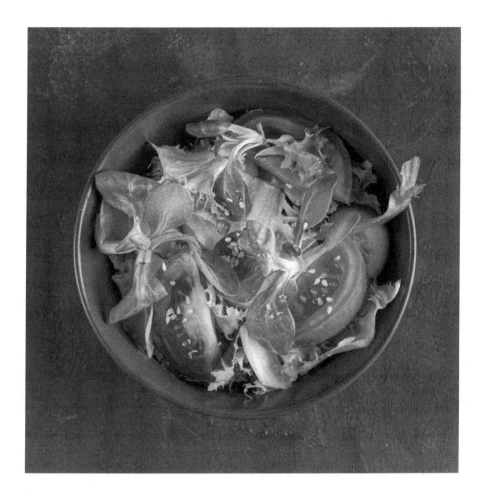

A fresh dinner can always be achieved through this fresh garden salad. The goodness of the salad is that it can serve as lunch, breakfast or dinner.

Servings: 4

Cook time: 1 minute

Ingredients:

- ¼ c. extra virgin olive oil
- ½ orange
- 1/3 c. black olives
- ½ orange juice
- ½ tsp. fine grain salt
- 1 handful salad greens, washed and dried
- ½ small purple onion, chopped
- ½ lemon juice

Directions:

1) Thoroughly mix salt, olive oil, red onion, lemon juice, and ½ of a juiced orange until you have an emulsified dressing. You can adjust lemon juice and salt according to your desired taste.

2) Cut and peel into segments the remaining orange half; set aside.

3) In a large salad bowl, arrange salad greens. Garnish with olives, onion, and orange segments. Pour dressing, and toss to coat.

4) Serve, and enjoy!

Greek Salad

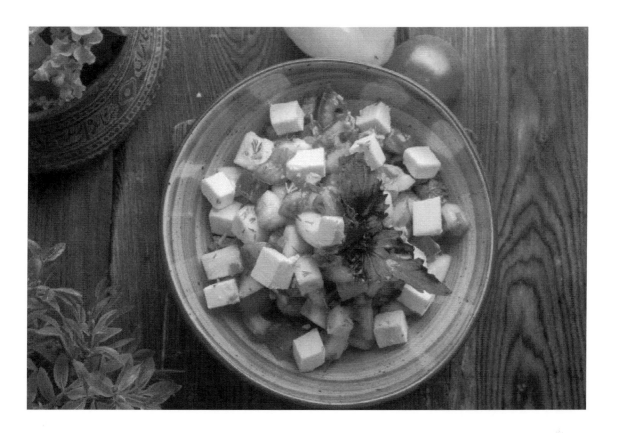

It is a wonderful quick salad prepared with a range of ingredients that are readily available. It is tasty and enjoyable.

Servings: 4

Cook time: 1 minute

Ingredients:

- ½ c. olive oil
- ½ medium-sized onion, thinly sliced
- 1 tbsp. dried oregano
- 2 garlic cloves, minced
- ½ purple onion, diced
- Pepper
- ½ lemon, juiced
- 1 English cucumber, diced
- 3 tomatoes, diced
- 1 red pepper, diced
- 1 tbsp. red wine vinegar

Directions:

1) Dice ingredients into uniform sizes, preferably ¼-½ inch cubes.

2) In a small bowl, mix dried oregano, vinegar, oil, sliced onion, and minced garlic, and set aside.

3) In a large bowl, mix onions, cucumbers, pepper, and tomatoes.

4) Pour in dressing, and toss to mix well before serving.

Braised Mushrooms and Swiss Chard

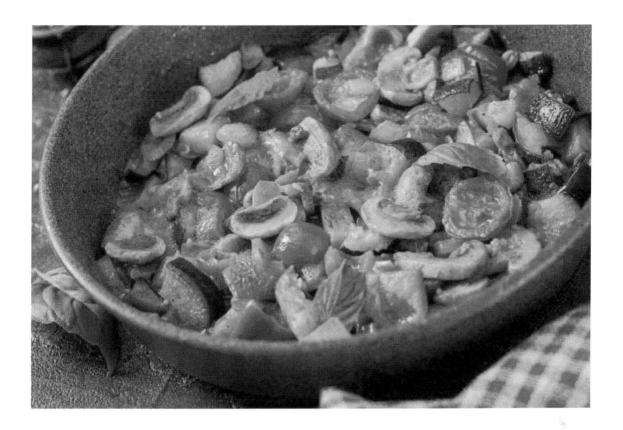

With Swiss Chard and mushrooms incorporated, you can be sure of the outstanding deliciousness of this recipe.

Servings: 4

Cook time: 5 minutes

Ingredients:

- 6 oz. shiitake mushroom, sliced ¼-inch thick
- 2 tbsp. unsalted butter
- 2 bunches Swiss chard, rinsed and dried, ribs removed and roughly chopped
- ¼ tsp. kosher salt

Directions:

1) On medium-high fire, place a large non-stick pan, and heat the butter.

2) Add mushrooms, and season with salt.

3) Only add chard once the mushrooms have given out their liquid.

4) Continue cooking while covered for around five minutes, while occasionally stirring.

5) Remove vegetables once cooked, and transfer to a serving plate to enjoy.

Lemon Chicken Grilled

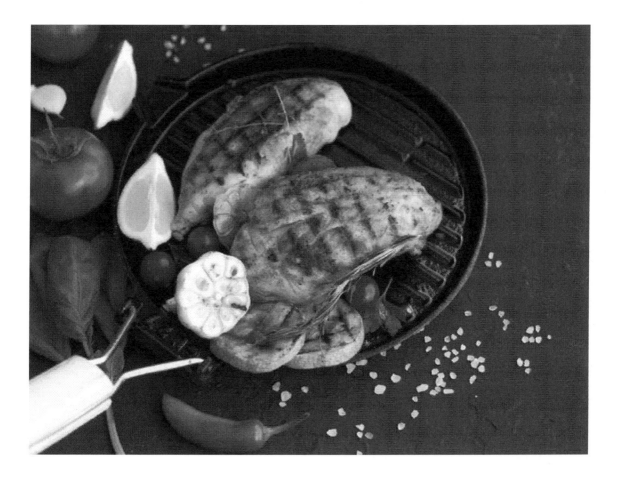

If you are now used to the normal way of preparing chicken, then you have to explore further. Your exploration should land you at this special meal. Enjoy the sweetness and the lemony taste.

Servings: 4

Cook time: 28 minutes

Ingredients:

- 2 large garlic cloves, finely chopped
- ¼ c. olive oil
- ¼ tsp. ground black pepper
- 2 tbsp. finely chopped red bell pepper
- 1/3 c. lemon juice
- ½ tsp. salt
- 4 skinless, boneless chicken breast halves
- 1 tbsp. Dijon mustard

Directions:

1) Combine pepper, salt, red bell pepper, garlic, Dijon mustard, olive oil, and lemon juice in a bowl, and mix well.

2) To use as basting, keep in a separate bowl ¼ of the liquid mixture.

3) Add chicken into the mixture, and allow the marinade to seep into the chicken for at least 20 minutes.

4) Oil the grate, and preheat the grill to high fire.

5) Once the grill is heated, add chicken, and cook for 6-8 minutes per side, or until juices run clear.

6) Every once in a while, baste the chicken with reserve marinade.

7) Once the chicken is cooked to the desired completion, remove it from the grill, and serve.

Skewered Bacon Ranch Chicken

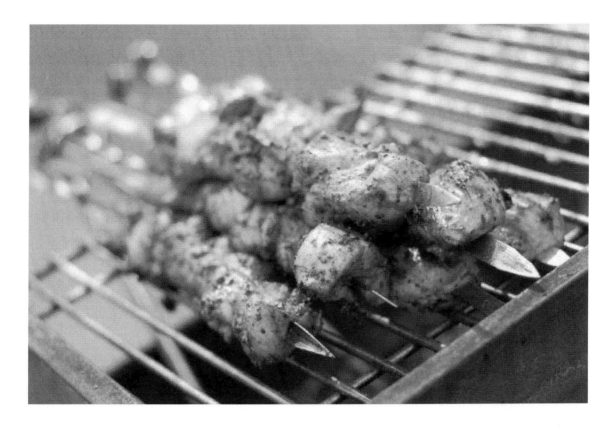

If you have to try out a unique dinner, then the skewered bacon ranch chicken should be your go-for meal. Enjoy it.

Servings: 12

Cook time: 10 minutes

Ingredients:

- 1/3 c. ranch dressing
- 12 pieces 6-inch long bamboo skewer, soaked for 2 hours
- 12 slices thick cut bacon
- 1 tsp. hot Chile paste
- 24 pieces 1-inch length red onions
- Pepper and salt
- 4 skinless, boneless chicken breast halves cut into 1-inch pieces

Directions:

1) In a large bowl, blend well hot Chile paste and ranch dressing. Toss in chicken to coat evenly, and allow to sit in the refrigerator for 1-3 hours.

2) Then, skewer chicken pieces and bacon by first threading in onion, then one end of a strip of bacon into the skewer. Then, add one chicken slice, and cover one side of chicken with bacon: thread bacon into skewer again. Repeat this around 4-5 times by adding 4-5 amounts of chicken and threading the bacon alternately like a letter S. Then, repeat the procedure until you have 12 skewered chicken and bacon.

3) Lightly oil the grate, and preheat grill to medium high fire.

4) Season with pepper, and salt the bacon/chicken skewers before placing them on the grill.

5) Grill each side for 3-4 minutes or until the meat is evenly browned and no longer pink.

6) Remove from grill, serve, and enjoy while hot.

Prime Rib with Garlic

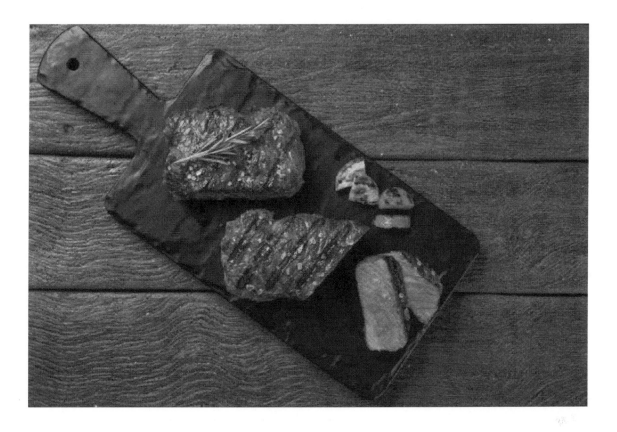

There is more deliciousness in this specially cooked prime rib. Regardless of whether it is expensive or not, you can go on extra miles to gauge its worthiness.

Servings: 6

Cook time: 1 hour 15 minutes

Ingredients:

- 2 tsp. salt
- 2 tsp. dried thyme
- 1 piece 10-lb prime rib roast
- 10 garlic cloves, minced
- 2 tsp. ground black pepper
- 2 tbsp. olive oil

Directions:

1) In a roasting pan, place roast on with the fatty side up.

2) Mix together thyme, pepper, salt, olive oil, and garlic in a small bowl.

3) Next, rub the herb mixture all over the roast, and let it sit at room temperature for an hour.

4) Preheat the oven to 500oF.

5) For twenty minutes, bake the rib roast on high fire to seal in the juice.

6) Lessen the temperature to 325oF and cool rib roast for 60-75 minutes. Ribs are done once the internal temperature of the roast has risen to 135oF.

7) Then, remove the roast from the oven. Let it rest for 10-15 minutes to retain its juice.

8) Carve the meat, serve, and enjoy.

Conclusion

Thank you again for downloading this book!

I hope you found valuable information from this book and ample encouragement to get started on the Dukan diet. Although it was initially deemed ineffective (without a strong scientific basis) by many dietitians and health experts, the Dukan diet is now proven effective with millions of people on its defense.

There are also many general practitioners and nutritionists who recommend the diet to many of their patients as they believe in its efficacy in stabilizing weight in the long term. With those said, there is virtually no reason not to try the Dukan diet today. It isn't only for weight loss per se but also for the betterment of your general health as well.

Thank you and good luck!

Author's Afterthoughts

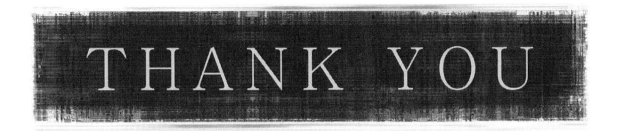

I am thankful for downloading this book and taking the time to read it. I know that you have learned a lot and you had a great time reading it. Writing books is the best way to share the skills I have with your and the best tips too.

I know that there are many books and choosing my book is amazing. I am thankful that you stopped and took time to decide. You made a great decision and I am sure that you enjoyed it.

I will be even happier if you provide honest feedback about my book. Feedbacks helped by growing and they still do. They help me to choose better content and new ideas. So, maybe your feedback can trigger an idea for my next book.

Thank you again

Sincerely

Ivy Hope

Printed in Great Britain
by Amazon